CAREGIVING
101

CAREGIVING
101

TAFFY CANNON

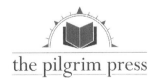

the pilgrim press

The Pilgrim Press, 700 Prospect Avenue East
Cleveland, Ohio 44115-1100
thepilgrimpress.com

© 2021 Taffy Cannon

All rights reserved. No part of this book may be used or reproduced in any manner
whatsoever without written permission.

Published 2021.

Printed on acid-free paper.
25 24 23 22 21   1 2 3 4 5

Library of Congress Cataloging-in-Publication Data on file.
LCCN: 2021943797
ISBN 978-0-8298-0640-3 (alk. paper)
ISBN 978-0-8298-0641-0 (ebook)
Printed in The United States of America.

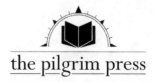

Book and cover design by Meredith Pangrace

This book is for all caregivers

– past, present, and future –

with love and respect

CONTENTS

INTRODUCTION

Nobody is ever ready.

You may be quietly preparing to care for a loved one who is becoming incapacitated. Or you may get the phone call that changes life in a millisecond.

Either way, you are embarking on a frightening journey through unfamiliar territory.

You may be dealing with disease, infection, accident, mental illness, or a raft of other conditions and illnesses that you've never even heard of before.

And something needs to be done. In fact, a lot of somethings probably need to be done. *Right now.*

I've been there.

My younger brother was just 51 when he suffered his first stroke, a long-delayed side effect of radiation treatment for a malignant brain tumor fourteen years earlier. He'd suffered numerous grand mal seizures in the intervening years, which resulted in cumulative brain damage. But the tumor had never returned, so we assumed we were out of the woods. We were wrong. We were just heading into a different part of the forest, one with no landmarks.

My brother was divorced, lived alone in Chicago, and had cut himself off from almost everyone. My sister was a veterinarian in Seattle and I was a writer in San Diego.

We were all clueless.

But we managed, and so can you.

This book is designed to help you sort out what needs to be done and determine what doesn't. Every situation is different and no two patients are alike, but there are certain common elements in all caregiving. We'll set those out and also offer options in situations that aren't so common.

The good news is that nobody needs all the information in this book. If you come across a section that has nothing to do with you, feel free to ignore it. You can also jump around as you need to and nobody will know or care.

When caregiving drops into your life, you can expect to experience a lot of different reactions, often one piled upon another. You may scream and yell. You will almost certainly cry. You're likely to lose track of everything you are doing. You may go onto autopilot at work. You may confront panic, or it may confront you.

And throughout all of this, you may secretly doubt that you will ever be able to handle all of the responsibility that has just been thrust upon you.

But remember that you are far from alone. Indeed, until becoming a caregiver, a lot of people don't even realize such a role exists, much less that caregivers form a widespread community.

So, hang on. You'll get through this. And you'll do it the same way you've managed the rest of your life: putting one foot in front of the other, doing the best you can, and hoping for the best.

ONE
First Steps: Evaluating the Situation

I t may feel as if you're slogging through quicksand when you first become immersed in caregiving. Here we'll help you find and narrow your focus, so you can deal more confidently with your individual situation.

Understanding the nature of your relationship to the patient, the type of medical problem they're facing, and what information is currently available about their diagnosis will put you on much firmer ground.

Which will help more than you might think.

Who's the Patient?

Not all caregiving situations are created equal, though the default is almost always family.

Yes, there is plenty of shared territory, but caring for a 97-year-old parent in a memory care unit is very different from caring for a 32-year-old child with cancer.

Always keep in mind that the patient is the most important part of the caregiving equation.

This seems obvious, but it can be easy to forget in times of crisis, when everybody gathers with lots of opinions.

If the patient is conscious and aware, it's important to include them in decision-making wherever possible. If you're lucky, they've already completed advance directives—legal paperwork that specifies the type of medical treatment they want and who gets to make decisions about it if they aren't able to (*see* CHAPTER FIVE: THE PAPER JUNGLE). If they haven't already completed advance directives, do everything possible to take care of this immediately.

Parents

Caregiving for parents of any age brings all manner of past issues and attitudes and problems and joys to the surface, in a jumble that increases exponentially when more than one child is involved.

Every child has a different relationship with every parent, and none of them are static. Your first-born brother knew very different parents in his early years as an only child than you did three kids down the line, a decade later.

Geography can be an issue here as well, particularly if your parent has retired to an inconvenient location.

Parents tend not to take easily to being told what to do and how to live by children who peed in their eye while their diapers were changed. They often have friends who have already been down this road and may have a better idea of what they *don't* want than what they do. They are likely to be in denial. They may be particularly resentful if you need to become involved in their financial affairs.

And they know exactly how to guilt-trip you from decades of experience.

Spouses

Caring for an ailing spouse has certain advantages, overbalanced by spectacular heartaches.

This is the one caregiving situation where you are there by choice, not accident of birth, and the one where you are most likely to really know how the other person ticks. Couples together for a long time may have all sorts of unrelated problems and unresolved issues, but in a serious health crisis those tend to be pushed aside, at least initially.

Keeping that baggage out of the way is important.

The word spouses here refers to any pair of people bound together by love and devotion, whether or not there is a legal union. Without a legal union, however, you may have problems, no matter how many years you've been together. HIPAA, the Health Insurance Portability and Accountability Act, was created in 1996 to protect patient privacy and limits who may have access to patient information. Getting the legal paperwork in order immediately is crucial.

Spouses usually start on the caregiving journey with a shared residence, which puts you ahead of the game, but also trapped inside it. You already know plenty about the patient's life, work, friends, activities, habits, irritations, and endearments. Your personal shorthand will serve as a foundation through what lies ahead.

Accept that you are not likely to make any changes to your partner or the previous dynamics of your relationship. If something changes significantly for any reason, including new and unfamiliar dependencies, try to roll with it and help your partner do the same as much as possible.

We're in this together is your motto, though living up to it won't always be easy.

Siblings

When you're caring for a sibling, it's generally because they don't already have some other sort of family support team in place. This may be through choice or circumstance, but it signals that your loved one is accustomed to doing things exactly the way they want to, usually while living alone.

Sibling relationships can range from sisters who speak on the phone every single day to the brother who hit the road at eighteen and never looked back. They may also bristle with unresolved past issues that have festered for decades.

An independent sibling may be extremely reluctant to accept help from anybody, no matter how much they need it. Geography can be a problem as well, since independent but suddenly needy siblings generally don't live just down the road.

You may not be able to help nearly as much as you would like. Or you may discover that you prefer not to be involved for any number of valid reasons. Some of these are absolute deal breakers, such as a history of sexual or other abuse.

Children

Caring for a child of any age with serious health problems may be the toughest challenge any parent will ever face. This is not what you envisioned on your path through parenthood, and it plays into everyone's primal fear of losing a child.

The age of the child is the governing factor here.

Adult children with serious health problems may be eager to fall back into the soft comfort of Mom or Dad's loving embrace. If that's what your kid wants, nothing is more important than to keep on hugging.

The urge to step in and help is instinctive, but feel your way cautiously. A parent (especially an opinionated and/or bossy one) can be a real pain. Even the best parent can get in the way if an adult child has their own strong established family unit. Divorced parents are a further complication.

Some adult children may not *want* to have their parents involved, in any combination or for any circumstance. That can be emotionally devastating. Remind yourself that you *did* raise them to be independent and self-sustaining adults, put a positive spin on it, and be warmly supportive in ways that your child appreciates. Send candy or fruit if there aren't dietary considerations, or flowers from time to time, or an item of clothing you're pretty sure they'd like.

Then back out of the way.

Parents of a young child with a major illness or injury face the most horrible and terrifying scenario possible.

This is worsened by people who have absolutely no idea what to do or say, and who almost invariably say the wrong things. Do your best to tune out this well-intentioned but horrible verbal clutter. If you want the physical comfort of a hug, murmur: "Just hugs, no talking." Feel free to burst into tears to shut them up.

If the doctor's office didn't bring it up right away, ask about local support groups. Parents of kids who have been through difficult health experiences are often willing—even eager—to help out somebody having a similar hard time.

Your child's terrible situation will also shake up your friends with young children. Some of them will withdraw out of not knowing what to say or do, plus a guilty awareness that they are relieved it was your child and not their own.

There is no positive side to this one.

Friends and Others

Most unpaid caregiving is family-based, but occasionally a situation arises where you are a logical caregiver for someone outside your own bloodlines. These tend to be highly specific and sometimes quite unusual setups.

There may be an older woman at church you've grown close to, somebody whose kids live off in Outer Nowhere. Or somebody who's lived independently for many years but is now on the cusp of having to make decisions about some kind of relocation. Your closest friend forever may be alone, or close to it. If that friend isn't nearby, you add the challenge of distance caregiving.

You might also become involved in caregiving by accident of geography if a neighbor needs transportation, yard work, or other assistance. This may be because their family members sought you out, or simply because you're a good person and the old guy's leaves needed raking.

SPRINT OR MARATHON?: CATEGORIES OF CAREGIVING

Most caregiving falls into one of the following categories: chronic and long-term, fast and deadly, short-term, or intermittent.

Identifying the one that applies to you may not solve anything, but it will ease you into a greater sense of control. A sense of control—even when fleeting—almost always helps.

Chronic and Long-Term

Chronic and long-term health situations may start out very differently, but much of the care and treatment runs along similar lines. Many involve deterioration over time.

This is what most people think of when they hear the term "caregiving."

Chronic health situations may meander for a while—sometimes for decades—before reaching crisis stage. Once properly diagnosed with a solid treatment plan, they are often extremely stable and manageable indefinitely with proper attention to medical detail.

All have the potential for a miracle drug to provide an outright cure or at least erase symptoms—though not necessarily this week, month, or year.

Diabetes is a classic instance of a chronic condition. So are multiple sclerosis, Parkinson's, and asthma.

However, these can also turn degenerative. Moving into this next stage and requiring assistance can be difficult to accept, particularly if the patient has successfully dealt with the problem for a long time.

Independence is very hard to relinquish.

Other long-term situations are more likely to explode into your life when you're least expecting them and to disrupt that life mightily.

Heart attacks, strokes, major accidents, head injuries—all cause instantaneous change for the patient and everyone around them. Ripples can spread quickly in many directions, and some are particularly difficult to control.

Denial usually crashes this party as well.

These patients may require vast amounts of treatment and rehabilitation, which may or may not be effective. This treatment only rarely returns a person to pre-event capabilities, especially if the brain is involved. Worst of all, the patient can't always register and accept the changes and new limitations, or communicate reactions to them.

A traumatic brain injury and a stroke may have dramatically different beginnings, but when the dust settles, patients of either one are likely to need lots of time, energy, and encouragement. What's more, both patients may be facing these new obstacles from a physical and/or mental level that is significantly diminished relative to their previous capabilities.

Alzheimer's and other forms of dementia are both chronic and long-term, making them even more difficult to deal with over time.

Chronic and long-term health conditions make a lot of demands on the caregiving team. One of these is awareness that the trajectory of the situation is probably downward, however slowly.

Caregiver burnout can build up just as slowly and steadily. That's dangerous for all concerned. You don't always have to be at your best, but you need to stay reasonably fresh. You absolutely need to step outside this caregiving world regularly.

Daily. No matter what the schedule, *take care of yourself* (*see* CHAPTER SEVEN: CARING FOR THE CAREGIVER).

Meanwhile, if you're a planner, it can help to back away a bit and at least try to answer these questions:

- What is likely to happen next?
- How will this affect my loved one's life?
- How will this affect *my* life?
- How long will this stage last?
- Will new treatment or medications be required?
- … and so on, and so on, and so on.

Fast and Deadly

Fast and deadly medical conditions are exactly what they sound like. They are dreadful in every possible way.

Malignant brain tumors are a classic example. AIDS used to be another. COVID-19 joined the club in 2020.

Some fast and deadly diseases actually take their own sweet time establishing themselves in a host's body before revealing themselves dramatically and/or after it's already too late to do much about them. Pancreatic and ovarian cancers are difficult to diagnose and even more difficult to treat.

It's extremely important to have a patient's legal paperwork in order in this type of situation (*see* CHAPTER FIVE: THE PAPER JUNGLE). Forcing this issue may be unpleasant, but it's essential. Do it.

Short-Term

Short-term caregiving situations are about as good as it gets.

They tend to be straightforward, with three rare features in the caregiving world: a beginning, a middle, and an end. They are sometimes optional, and often emergencies. There's a specific goal that everybody understands in advance and hospital stays are brief.

Minor accidents fall into this category, along with most elective surgeries. Joint replacements provide some of the happiest examples.

Best of all, the patient almost always feels better when it's over.

Intermittent

In some intermittent medical situations, an illness such as MS flares up periodically. Or a back injury seems to be better until it isn't. Here you need to address both the immediate problem and its potential for future trouble.

A lot of cancer therapies are intermittent—scheduled for definite durations at prolonged intervals. Chemotherapy and radiation both require very specific protocols and schedules. Accordingly, caregiving and transport also require serious scheduling.

It's limited comfort, but there's one distinct advantage to intermittent caregiving: When a medical situation repeats itself predictably, you will be knowledgeable and experienced the next time around.

WHAT'S GOING ON?

That's the central question in all caregiving, and the answer changes all the time. At some points you may be asking this question on an hourly basis. Later you may look for signs of improvement after onerous treatments, a process that can spread out over weeks and months. In the case of dementia, the mental decline you are tracking may be relatively slow or distressingly fast.

The most significant information to track, at least initially, is the patient's evolving medical condition.

Often in your heart of hearts you really don't want to know what's going on. Many of the answers are likely to be bad, or at least discouraging. Prayer can help. It is also perfectly all right to lock yourself in a room and scream yourself hoarse or overindulge yourself in some uncharacteristic way.

If you haven't been around for the prelude to this medical situation, you'll need to track down whatever you can about previous treatments, testing, and medication—usually in conjunction with the primary care physician or somebody who's been involved in the patient's care.

Don't assume that you already know what's going on, even if you live with the patient or have spoken regularly during the lead-up to the diagnosis. You can easily have missed something.

Sometimes the problem is that there *weren't* any medical complaints and should have been because the patient was ignoring symptoms.

A lot of people who fear that they have a serious or life-threatening illness prefer to ignore it and hope that one day they'll wake up cured. And if the medical complaint is embarrassing in some way, people are even more inclined to tough it out until they simply can't ignore symptoms any longer.

Understanding the Disease

It's an excellent idea to do some basic research into the immediate medical situation.

The internet is your close personal friend in this quest for medical information, so long as you keep a few rules in mind.

When you Google a disease, you'll get a list of hits that generally starts out with half a dozen places that would like you to come to their facility for treatment. Skip all of them for now. Also ignore any ads that come up, particularly the ones that assure you of an easy cure.

Look first for a foundation devoted to the diagnosed disease.

Sometimes there will be several. You may need to dig a little: look for information or links buried within a major foundation's website, such as stroke at the American Heart Association or lymphedema at the American Cancer Association.

When you locate the appropriate disease website, sign up for any relevant online mailing lists. There are usually other ways to get more information, including calling an 800 number the old-fashioned way. These lines are answered by people who are knowledgeable and caring, and they understand how difficult it can be to even say the nature of the problem out loud. They may be able to offer information on support groups in your area and can almost certainly provide literature by snail mail.

You can find tons of books online—enough to keep you so busy reading that you won't have time to take care of the patient. Ration the information you try to absorb and don't push yourself beyond what you actually need to know at any particular point.

Harvard Medical School Special Reports provide concise, clear, and current information about anything that might be wrong with anybody. If you want a reference for a specific situation or condition, start here.

Definitely do collect information about your loved one's diagnosis from the people involved in their medical care: doctors, nurses, technicians, therapists. But also understand that these people may have limited time, or questionable people skills, or not enough information about the specifics of this particular diagnosis. Somebody who knows a lot about nutrition in cancer treatment may not know much about multiple myeloma.

Looking for Answers

Sometimes there aren't any answers.

This can be difficult to accept. You want the cure that nobody has found yet, or improved treatment from what's been done for twenty years, or an answer to the most agonizing question of all: *Why?*

Most people do spend a fair amount of time thinking and talking about *Why?* Sometimes it seems obvious, like a lifelong smoker contracting lung cancer or a person who consumes a lot of carbohydrates developing diabetes. But people who've behaved perfectly and eaten healthy also get lung cancer and diabetes.

The reality is that it no longer matters.

Why? is tough to let go of, however, and sometimes the patient has the hardest time. If somebody keeps bringing this up, develop conversational ploys to deflect the question and change the subject as quickly as possible.

How about those Cowboys/Dodgers/Bulls?

Sharing Information Online

Sharing information with those who want or need to know can be difficult, especially if you are in a new and complicated medical situation. Very few people enjoy telling the same sad story over and over and over again, but in an electronic age that really isn't necessary.

By all means speak personally with the folks you normally talk to, but find other information pathways as well.

If the circle to be informed is relatively small, you may be able to keep everybody informed with group texts or emails. If it's mostly Luddites, revert to the old-fashioned telephone tree, but remember that it only takes one unresponsive branch or broken twig to render any communication incomplete or inaccurate.

Often a number of people are interested and concerned, but not necessarily actively involved. To facilitate keeping them informed, consider setting up a personal website with *caringbridge.org*.

CaringBridge is free and it's designed to let you share information easily. When you (or your tech support nephew) set up the patient's website, you can decide how much information is included, who gets to add material, and when and how to share new developments. You can even set up a way for people to share good wishes with the patient.

Control privacy levels carefully. Where caregiving and social media intersect, less is almost always more.

Be very wary of putting any health care information onto social media without the patient's express permission. No, not just permission—enthusiasm. If you know that the patient would be horrified to have her hospital picture on Facebook hooked up to IVs and machinery, then don't even consider it.

The Exception That Proves the Rule

There is one type of information that you absolutely do not want.

That's the unsolicited account from the person whose relative or close friend had exactly what your family member has now and had the world's worst time with it. These folks turn up everywhere.

They genuinely believe that they are helping. But these stories don't tend to end with butterflies fluttering on a soft summer day while everybody lives happily ever after. They are much more likely to involve dismemberment, hideous side effects, horrible drug reactions, gargantuan medical bills, possible malpractice, worsening conditions and, of course, death.

Cut these people off as quickly as you can.

If this is somebody you see frequently, just say, *I'm sorry, but I really need to save your story for another time. I'm sure you understand.* You may need to repeat this several times. Practice saying it in front of a mirror until it becomes less uncomfortable. Feel free to burst into tears if somebody simply will not let up.

If it's somebody you don't see often, it's even easier. *I'm sorry, but I'm too distressed to talk right now. Keep us in your thoughts and prayers.* Then make your departure during the consoling statements that follow.

In either case, move purposefully on your way. You aren't being rude. You're protecting your own mental health.

TWO
GETTING ORGANIZED

How you approach this critical element of caregiving will reflect how you feel about the concept of organization in general.

If you know the location of every Q-tip and can of corn in your house and regularly dust the linen closet, you have probably already taken care of a lot of these details.

However, if you approach organizing anything with dread and hate hearing people's cheery reports about how happy they are now that they have gotten rid of everything that was in the garage, you are going to need to bite some bullets here.

Do it. Get started. A lot of these things simply can't wait.

SUPPORT FOR THE PATIENT AND THE CAREGIVER

Sometimes everybody agrees about everything. If this is your family's situation, congratulations. You may be in a difficult and unhappy place, but at least you're all rowing in the same direction.

Once you accept that you are on the caregiving path, it's critical to gather two things: a support system and detailed information about the patient and their medical issues.

In addition, if you are assuming responsibility for such non-medical tasks as personal finance, you can't wait too long to dig in. Your world may be in chaos, but the bills still need to be paid.

Seeking Support

Learn how to ask for help.

Babies instinctively know how to do this, initially through crying and then through smiling, language, and physical gestures.

Unfortunately, that instinct dissipates in many people, and by the time some folks reach their seventh or eighth decades, it may have all but disappeared.

If you are one of those people, you need to learn how to adjust your ways. Caregiving is hard, hard work. The hours are long and the rewards limited. When you are a primary caregiver, even for the saintliest soul, you need all the help you can get.

In addition, some people are particularly independent— sometimes to the point of pigheadedness. They can take care of everything on their own, thank you very much.

If the patient is excessively independent, it's quite possible that medical and other matters were already in an advanced stage by the time you got involved. The patient may not have requested help at all and might feel put-upon and angry because help was thrust upon them.

At this point you have a lot less chance of changing the patient than of changing your own behavior, at least temporarily. If you are *both* ultra-independent, just grit your teeth and get used to the idea that for now you're going to have to ask for help.

You won't regret it.

Patients Who Just Want to Be Left Alone

This is a tough one.

Here you are, ready and willing to help in any way you can, and your loved one wants nothing to do with you, your attentions, or any other part of this developing medical mess. It can help here to try to put yourself in the patient's place.

When you are sick or injured or otherwise incapacitated, everything in your world gets twisted and turned and tied in knots.

For many patients—and some caregivers!—the first response is to pull the covers over their head, and just wait until it gets better. This is a perfectly reasonable reaction and one that almost anybody can identify with, at least initially. After a while, most folks will snap—or at least crawl—out of this funk.

The last thing a withdrawing patient wants is to be surrounded by jolly folks offering chicken soup and well-wishes and advice.

While you're getting started, work around this patient as much as you can. Take care of whatever you can without getting in the patient's face or business any more than absolutely necessary. Figure out what must be done and insist that the patient attempt to cooperate.

With time, the patient may not be any happier, but you probably won't need to tiptoe quite so much.

Who's the Advocate?

When you are really sick and incapacitated, it's important to be on top of what is wrong with you and what can be done to make it better. But you are also less likely to be able to take on this responsibility yourself.

The solution is an advocate. Every patient needs one.

As early as possible, you should identify and designate one or more advocates to cover such responsibilities as medical matters, creditors, and insurance or other disputes.

This advocate may or may not be you. There is no dishonor in passing on the responsibility to somebody more comfortable being assertive in difficult situations. The advocate responsibilities may also be best divided among a combination of people with special skills and special relationships with the patient. That's all fine.

First and foremost, you need somebody to pay attention to the medical details.

If the patient is hospitalized, this advocate needs to keep track of who's doing what, and what is or isn't scheduled, and what's happening next and why. As time goes by, a medical advocate will accompany the patient to medical appointments, keep track of the loose ends, schedule necessary supplemental or referral appointments, and ask the hard questions.

An advocate needs to make sure that the patient's needs and questions are addressed every step of the way.

An advocate may also need to be the bad guy who takes on unresponsive medical personnel or recalcitrant insurance companies, using a combination of persistence, attention to detail, and charm.

Building a Support Team

One of the many ironies of caregiving is that when you least know what is going on or where it is headed, people are most likely to offer help.

They usually mean it, too. But most folks aren't trained or skilled at caregiving, so they may be as clueless as you are about creating your caregiving support team. Building that team is a challenge, but well worth the time and effort.

Remember that caregiving covers a lot of territory. It isn't just offering tea to a bedridden patient wearing a lacy peignoir. In fact, it almost never is.

It can include cooking or cleaning or yard work or clearing gutters or hanging up the Christmas lights. Walking the dog, re-configuring the furniture, building a ramp, diving into a tangled financial morass.

The particulars vary from one case to another, but there almost always is more involved than simple patient care.

Which is, of course, never simple.

Just who should be included in the caregiving support team?

Start with anybody who already has a close personal relationship with the patient.

Immediate family will usually be front and center, at least at the beginning. This provides an opportunity to assess how useful—or challenging—they are going to be, particularly with familial wild cards.

Everybody else comes next, in no particular order.

This may include parents, children of any age, friends, neighbors, clergy, fellow parishioners, former spouses, coworkers—or all of these swirled into a slightly confusing stew. Don't forget the men who fish together in the summer, the women who knit on Tuesdays, fellow volunteers, the book club, and the folks from the VFW.

You probably already know some of these people and may have heard about some of the others. Nobody will expect you to know them all, even if the patient is your spouse.

If they're local and you're in the middle of a *SURPRISE!* crisis such as a stroke or automobile accident, they may be involved already: visiting the hospital, making airport runs, bringing meals, asking how they can help.

It's a little different when a situation has arisen over time, perhaps through a series of troubling but unexplained medical problems, or through growing memory issues. Finally getting an answer can be both a relief and a nightmare. On the one hand, you can finally focus on dealing with what's wrong. On the other hand, it's cancer or dementia.

Often friends or relatives have been involved through this process of Figuring It Out, so they are already on hand to help with what needs to be done. That helps a lot.

Spend some time thinking about how people can actually help and give specific assignments if you possibly can.

This will (a) get stuff done and (b) create a community of people who have helped once and are therefore more likely to help again.

Your job is to make specific assignments: *Go to the store and get more half-and-half. Pick up a bag of burgers for dinner. Take the dog to the vet. Take the dog to* your *house for a few days. Gas my car up. We're out of cat litter. Fold the laundry. Pick up and get rid of all the throw rugs.*

Pay attention to who's around, whether they're helpful or not, and get *everybody's* contact information.

This is easiest at the beginning. You have no way of knowing who you might want or need later, and it's natural to ask for contact info early on. Scraps of paper are fine, or business cards for those who have them. Toss them all in the contacts bin (see below in "The Patient's Permanent Record").

If you're looking for help with hands-on caregiving, sound out prospects about their experience and make the questions open-ended. *What did you do when you helped care for your mother?* may expand the discussion into areas you haven't even thought of yet. And the answer may also reveal that somebody will be more trouble than they are worth.

Sickroom care isn't always easy and it's usually not for the faint-hearted. If even thinking about the basics of commodes and changing wound dressings and wiping fevered brows is beyond your comfort zone, look for others who may be better suited.

You may need to hire help in some cases, either right away or down the road. Unless you are very well-to-do, this isn't a logical or easy first choice.

For intimate care such as bathing and bathroom assistance, offer the patient plenty of input. Just because somebody is eager to help or the patient likes them a lot doesn't necessarily mean that they want their help getting on and off the pot.

As the situation becomes clearer, you'll begin to realize what you actually do need. Maybe dinner a couple of times a week, or rides to radiation, or watching the kids after school, or walking the dogs, or raking the leaves, or spending time with the patient while you do something else, like take a nap.

Transportation can be helpful in all kinds of ways, whether it's airport pickups, prescription fetching, or Thursday rides to physical therapy. Some of these tasks may involve scheduling. If this isn't one of your strong suits, find somebody on the team who loves lists and spreadsheets and calendars. Have them do it.

If there's a lot of scheduling involved, arrange for backups in case somebody wakes up with sniffles and a fever on the day they're supposed to drive to chemo.

Flexibility Is Key

Flexibility is your new best friend, even if it's not a natural behavior for you.

You are likely to discover that something you thought was going to be important or complicated actually isn't. Or that something you never even considered actually is.

At every juncture, be prepared for surprises, and willing to change your plans. If something doesn't work, scrap it. If somebody suggests something that sounds promising, listen.

If you're a planner by nature, your inclination will be to look ahead and try to prepare for what's next. This is logical and useful and sometimes it works. However, try not to plan too far ahead. Caregiving situations can change fast, sometimes in totally unanticipated directions.

Strive for a balance between winging it and creating full-fledged battle plans.

Difficult People

Let's take a moment to confront an unfortunate reality in many families: difficult people.

Difficult people come in all shapes, sizes, and styles. They can be difficult in endlessly different and annoying ways.

They don't always know they are being difficult. In fact, they often wouldn't believe it, because a certain level of obstinacy tends to move in tandem with this behavior—along the lines of: *Well, of course I'm right.* Difficult behaviors can also run in families, which you already know if you are nodding your head right now.

Do your best to defuse any kind of negative energy if you possibly can.

If there's a specific problem among certain participants, first appeal to their better natures, and if that doesn't work do your best to keep them apart. You don't have time to deal with this nonsense just now.

Maybe there are tasks the difficult person(s) can do to help that don't involve being around all the time. Online medical research? Dog walking? Bill paying? Grocery shopping? Getting the oil changed? It is also perfectly all right to create make-work chores to keep these folks occupied elsewhere, like over in the next county.

If communication with the difficult person is part of the problem, build in a little distance by primarily using email and text. That also creates a record.

Be prepared for a particularly challenging caregiving journey if the patient is the difficult one.

Faith-Based Communities

If the patient is part of a faith-based community of any sort, you may already have a built-in support group.

Most religious communities have some level of coordinated help mechanisms for situations just like yours. Maybe they bring meals or provide rides to medical appointments. Clergy may visit, along with deacons or other laity involved in the church's mission of doing good and caring for its own.

Whether or not this is your own faith community, you should work with these good folks the best you are able. People who genuinely care provide a comfort that can't be faked or purchased. Say *Thank you* often and mean it.

The perfect caregiving situation might comprise an entire group of people who are members of the same denomination or, even better, the same church. Everybody here will be on pretty much the same religious page. And if the patient is active and/or beloved in the religious community, the level of help offered usually increases.

You could end up with a freezer full of casseroles for quite some time.

Support Groups

There are basically two kinds of support groups: in person and online. These exist for various combinations of caregivers, relatives, and patients.

They can be lifelines, and you absolutely want to seek them out.

Support groups can be a great source of information as well as comfort and encouragement. The earlier you become involved in some of these, the better. People in health care support groups are down there in the trenches with you, and the solace and assistance you provide one another can be invaluable.

Not everybody is ready for this at the same time, and often patients are the most reluctant. Somebody with a strong healthy self-image may not be ready to brand themselves just yet with the name of a horrible disease, not to mention admitting to strangers what they are having trouble admitting to themselves: that they have a very serious health problem.

How do you find a support group? You may be able to find one that meets in person through the hospital or medical facility you are using. A lot of these places also have social workers who can steer you in the right direction or perhaps provide other contacts or info.

Senior centers and churches often have support groups related to Alzheimer's and dementia.

In-person support groups have some special advantages. Because the participants are local, they are likely to know about services and facilities and medical providers in your area. Are you looking for a second opinion? A fresh perspective? Holistic information? Somebody is likely to know about this, or to know somebody else who will know.

You aren't expected to know anything when you arrive, and usually people will be warm and welcoming. You may not be able to easily discuss your own situation, but you're likely to pick up useful nuggets even if you never open your mouth.

You may find one or more to be a poor fit for you and your current needs. If they are dealing with a different stage of an illness, particularly a later and less optimistic stage, your enthusiastic optimism about beating this may feel a bit out of line. If that's the case, don't go back, and don't feel guilty that it didn't work.

Foundations related to the disease or problem may also help you find an in-person support group in your area. Regrettably, this is more likely if the health problem you are dealing with is widespread.

Foundations are also an excellent source for online support groups, which may prove more useful, particularly if the medical problem is somewhat out of the ordinary. If you've never heard of this disease before, the likelihood of finding a dozen locals with the same problem isn't great. But if you connect with the right group online, you might get great information from people in Boise, Tampa, and Bangor, all in the same day.

The best sources for online support groups vary over time, and much of the current sharing action is on Facebook. These Facebook support groups are usually private and moderated. That means that only people who have been vetted for eligibility by a moderator are allowed to participate, and that posts may also be passed through a filter before going public.

Public in this sense does not mean the whole wide world. Yes, there's a ton of hacking and viruses and other online misbehaviors, but most people are entirely comfortable posting in online groups on social media. If you aren't sure about the privacy levels, check first with the moderator, and if there isn't a moderator, head for the hills.

Online support groups run through disease foundations may have different posting mechanisms and protocols. If this prospect confuses or frightens you, have somebody who is comfortable with this kind of online interaction set things up for you.

There's also nothing to stop you from setting up your own impromptu support group.

Take Care of Yourself
(*see* Chapter 7: Caring for the Caregiver)

This is the single most important piece of advice in this book: Take care of yourself.

Whether you ease into caregiving or it explodes into your life, it will complicate that life. Guaranteed.

A lot of these complications are things that you might never have thought about before, so there's also a pretty steep learning curve, with a few unmarked twists here and there. Any time you think you've actually worked something out, it's likely to change.

So adapt, and adapt some more, and soldier on.

Over time, this soldiering begins to take tolls that you might not initially recognize.

Sleep deprivation or insomnia or both. Getting behind on your own stuff. Altering meal habits for yourself as well as the patient. Problems at work. Missing events. Weight gain or weight loss. Normal nuisances becoming major obstacles: laundry, dishes, shoveling snow.

Levels of anxiety careening right off the charts.

From the very beginning, make sure to do at least one nice thing for yourself every single day.

It doesn't need to be big or dramatic. You may not yet have time for that sort of thing anyway. But it needs to happen.

Five minutes for sure, ideally twice a day. Fifteen if things are going smoothly or you have a little momentary relief. Take a walk around the block, sans cell phone. Move into a corner with your music device and earbuds, listening to personal music that soothes you or energizes you or maybe both. Even a shower or a brief bubble bath can be a lifesaver.

Stay in touch with your own friends and let them support you. If you didn't already realize this, you'll probably discover that some of them have had their own caregiving experiences. They get it.

Meet up at your place or the patient's or somewhere else altogether, like a restaurant or the nail salon or the library. Get the hot fudge sundae.

After a while, this self-care should become a habit, and it's a mighty useful one.

THE PATIENT'S PERMANENT RECORD

Childhood's eternal threat: *This is going to go on your permanent record.*

And yet, even when it *did* go on your permanent record, it mostly didn't matter much, and after a while, everybody forgot about it.

As a caregiver, you need to compile a very different sort of permanent record, one that actually matters a lot. Much of this will seem intrusive—because it is. Not all of it will be necessary in every situation. Some things are vital and others not so much. And you will, of course, be doing a few hundred other things at the same time.

Sorting out what you need to know is the first step.

Patient Information

These are the patient basics you'll need all the time, for every single form you fill out. Assemble all of this info as quickly as possible:

- Full legal name
- Address
- Phone number(s)
- Date of birth
- Email address(es)
- Social Security number
- Medicare number
- Health insurance company name and policy number

Photocopy any cards with this info, front and back.

Even if the patient can't help, the process should still be relatively simple. It may involve no task more complicated than opening the patient's wallet.

Print a copy of the basic info for your own wallet and create a digital version to store on your computer, phone, and/or other devices. You need this info at the ready even if you have the world's best memory and are sure you won't forget anything.

When you have legal paperwork such as advance directives or power of attorney (*see* CHAPTER 5: THE PAPER JUNGLE), you should also carry those on the phone or device, because the one time you forget the paperwork will naturally be the one time you really need it.

If the patient does not already have a current government-issued driver's license or ID, do your best to get one ASAP, usually through the state Department of Motor Vehicles. Expired IDs don't count. REAL ID requirements have made this process more complicated.

Contacts

This is a hodgepodge of all the people and organizations and agencies you are involved with in the pursuit of the patient's welfare. It includes relatives, doctors, therapists, technicians, friends, coworkers, clergy, household service people, and neighbors.

Business cards are the easiest way to do this. Take at least two and save one for the medical notebook (discussed below). If there's no card, write down the person's name, phone, email, and buzzwords to remind you why you might need the information. (Old friend, accountant, church deacon, etc.) You may never need or want much of this information, but collect it all now when it's easy.

Put these cards and scraps of paper into a small contacts container, such as a basket, box, or bin, and keep it accessible. It doesn't need to be orderly. Indeed, that's part of its charm.

Master Notebook

The rest of the medical information you collect belongs in a master notebook that is as comprehensive as possible. Much of this information is intrusive and highly personal.

It doesn't need to be widely distributed, nor should it be. The patient may fight tooth and nail against assembling it at all. Stand your ground and promise to have a bonfire when the patient is fully recovered and it's no longer necessary. Cross your fingers if recovery is problematic.

You need this information, and you need it now.

Start with a three-ring binder and a set of dividers. Get a pack of three-ring paper and/or a three-ring punch for computer-generated materials. You'll want some dividers with pockets or page protectors into which you can put loose or fragile pieces of relevant paper. Some of these will zip or snap closed. Any office supply store has all of this.

The master notebook brings together medical history, current medications, current medical information, health care providers, personal dossier, medical billing, and financial information.

Medical History

This can be extraordinarily complicated or breathtakingly simple, depending on the patient.

If the patient prided themself on never going to the doctor, everybody in the caregiving equation is pretty much starting from scratch. You'll learn what needs to be included as you head down the medical yellow brick road.

A younger patient may have no real medical history at all. Young adults are often lax about regular medical checkups, Pap smears, or anything beyond visiting the emergency room when weekend sports go awry. These are the kids who don't follow up ER treatment with their primary care physician because they aren't even sure what that is.

As a general rule, the older the patient, the more complicated the medical history will be. Sorting out which parts are important may take a while, and things that happened long ago may only be relevant if there is a particularly difficult diagnostic process.

Maintain perspective. It doesn't really matter whether a seventy-year-old was thirty-five or forty for his appendectomy, but it's important to know that he has experienced intermittent intense headaches for several years.

If a primary concern is dementia or other forms of memory loss, the patient may not be able to help much in reconstructing a medical history. Do the best you can.

If somebody has a reputation as a hypochondriac (deserved or otherwise) it can be tricky to sort out which medical complaints are legitimate. Just remember that even hypochondriacs can get really, really sick.

This is what you want to document in the medical history:

- All current diagnoses
- Physicians consulted in the past five years
- OB/GYN history for women
- Surgeries
- Any major medical problems, even if resolved long ago
- Significant past injuries
- Relevant past medications, such as antidepressants

Current Medications

This sounds easy, but it actually changes all the time in many medical situations, particularly new ones.

Keep the records current, and also put the list on your phone or tablet for reference. It can be useful to have it on the refrigerator or the inside door of the bathroom medicine cabinet, too, especially if the patient lives alone or has memory issues. Usually, it's a good idea to combine this with a pill dispenser to simplify matters (*see* CHAPTER 4: DIAGNOSIS, TREATMENT, AND MEDICATION).

The current medications list should include:

- Full medication names (not "blood pressure pills"), including *all* vitamins and supplements
- Dosages
- What the medication is taken for
- Prescribing physician
- Pharmacy where it is filled
- How often the medication is taken or applied

In some cases, this will create a hefty document—all the more reason to set it up.

If the patient is seeing a number of different specialists in different facilities, coordinating meds is critical. For starters, not everyone may have access to the same electronic records and information.

It is vitally important for every health care provider to know every current medication. This allows them to prescribe meds that will work and play well with each other. Carry the list to all appointments and make sure that anybody prescribing anything sees it. Every time.

Medications can interact badly with one another, up to and including death. We've all heard the voice-overs on those TV commercials for fancy new (expensive) drugs.

If ordering meds in three-month sets is an option to save money, wait to order three-months' worth until you're sure this is going to be a long-term medication. Some medications just don't work out, for all sorts of reasons. You don't want to get stuck with something pricey that you don't need.

Current Medical Information

This will be ongoing, and includes all kinds of paperwork: lab results, pathology reports, radiology reports, and any regularly scheduled treatments.

Start with the current treatment plan and the projected treatment plan if there is one.

Organize this section however works best for the situation. If you're tracking something in particular (pulse and blood pressure, for instance) here's the place to keep the chart.

Create charts with a spreadsheet program if that's in your skill set, or with a pen and ruler if it isn't. You can also download and print free blank monthly calendars.

Keep track of scheduled events both electronically and on an old-fashioned calendar with big-enough daily squares, and make sure that everybody who needs the information has access to it.

If the patient is part of any large-scale health care system, there may be an electronic system for patients to get immediate information about appointments, lab work, and much more from any computer or device.

For obvious reasons, access to this info is carefully controlled, and the patient may need to sign a form to give you access. You might also need to set it up if the patient hasn't done so previously.

It's worth the trouble for the convenience.

Health Care Providers

Pick up two business cards for every doctor, therapist, treatment center, and pharmacy you use. Put one in the contacts bin (discussed above) and keep another taped or stapled to a page in the medical notebook. Leave enough space to be able to make notes or comments, such as *out-of-network*, or *very rude*, or *came from Boston*. Don't forget Medicaid info, Medicare Supplement (Medigap) or Advantage plan contacts, and pharmacies, both local and mail order.

Include any information sources you have found helpful, such as disease information websites and support groups, along with any necessary login information.

Personal Dossier

This non-medical area becomes immediately intrusive. However, it's really important if you're dealing with somebody who is seriously ill or disabled, or on the road to being either.

Begin by assembling all the personal information in the "Patient Information" section above—the patient's basic name, rank, and serial number. Then augment it with additional info and documents. Photocopies are fine for now. You want:

- Marriage and divorce records with dates
- Military records with dates and discharge papers
- Passport
- Residency, citizenship, and naturalization papers if applicable
- Copies of legal documents that deal with specific medical and financial situations, including advance directives, will, and power of attorney (names for these vary from state to state, as we'll discuss in CHAPTER FIVE: THE PAPER JUNGLE)
- Info on *all* insurance policies, including health, dental, vision, life, disability, automobile, property, excess or umbrella, long-term care, and anything out of the ordinary, such as veterinary care. Include policy numbers, websites, phone numbers, and contact info for the company and any facilitating agent. How often are they paid and how? Direct debit, check, electronically?
- Passwords! You may need these to share information on social media on the patient's behalf, or to pay bills, or to gain info about … well, about anything and everything. Be prepared for resistance in sharing them with you and emphasize that the patient can change them all immediately when the medical crisis ends.

Current Medical Bills and Receipts

These don't need to be in the master notebook, but they should all be in one place, ideally in folders or large envelopes. Label these clearly, either by provider name or by category: paid, unpaid, disputed, hospital, out-of-network, whatever.

Disputes and issues arise constantly related to medical bills and it generally isn't because insurance paid more than you were expecting. If you have to fight with providers or insurance companies, it's extremely important to have all the information readily available.

You can fine tune the organization of this paperwork while you wait on hold.

Financial Information

This may be totally unnecessary if you're dealing with a spouse and you are the one who handles the money. If you're dealing with a parent or sibling or adult child, you may have difficulty getting access to a lot of this information on the grounds that it is none of your business.

Which normally it wouldn't be.

If you do need to be involved in financial matters and decisions, keep the information you accumulate for this purpose both secure and entirely separate from the medical info you've assembled. More detailed material about finances comes in CHAPTER FIVE: THE PAPER JUNGLE.

Wherever possible, include login information to relevant websites, as well as contact information for various agents and advisors and attorneys and accountants and counselors and administrators. Most of these will require some kind of written permission from the patient if you don't have power of attorney.

Here's what you may find you need. If a category doesn't apply, ignore it.

- Power of attorney
- Bank information: accounts, locations, login numbers, PINs
- Signatory on bank accounts
- All sources of income, including untapped sources such as pensions or Social Security
- Credit card info (photocopy cards front and back)
- Automobile or other vehicular payments
- Recurring bills paid automatically
- Safe deposit box locations and key whereabouts
- Real property, including land, houses, cars, boats, planes, RVs, motorcycles, ATVs, snowmobiles, farm machinery, and anything else with wheels and an engine
- Jewelry
- Art
- Investments, including stocks, bonds, savings accounts, credit unions, and IRA and 401K accounts

THREE
MEDICAL PERSONNEL AND FACILITIES

A lmost any situation that involves caregiving also involves interaction with the medical world.

Most caregiving involves a great deal of that interaction. Nothing is going to make that interaction easy, but it's important to figure out who you are dealing with and what these people do. The same is true for all kinds of medical facilities, and you may be surprised to discover just how many of those exist.

WHO'S WHO IN THE MEDICAL WORLD

The medical world used to be simple and straightforward: doctors and nurses.

The doctors were men and the nurses were women.

Today more women than men are enrolled in medical schools and the gender breakdown among younger doctors inches toward fifty-fifty. The move toward gender parity is far slower for nursing, however. A hundred years ago, only one percent of nurses were male; today about thirteen percent of nursing students are men.

Both inside and outside the traditional doctor-nurse framework, matters get more complicated.

Doctors

Doctors are at the top of the medical pecking order, and they like it that way.

They make the diagnoses and decisions, the treatment recommendations and prescriptions for pharmaceuticals. They poke, probe, query, investigate, evaluate, test, and evaluate some more. They oversee actual treatment, whether they are personally dispensing it or not.

These are huge responsibilities, and doctors know it.

As the daughter of a surgeon, I can tell you that the legend of the doctor-with-the-God-complex is based on hard, cold reality.

Which makes a certain amount of sense, because the doctoring business *does* involve life-or-death decisions, complicated investigations, and treatments that might go amiss without warning. When they get it right—and for the most part all doctors do—they are indeed carrying out functions that may be considered God-like.

One reason for this sense of superiority is the extraordinary competition to enter this line of work. It is incredibly difficult to become a doctor in the United States, and many more highly qualified young people want to be doctors than slots are available to accommodate them.

It may be difficult to determine how good a doctor is. People tend to rate their physicians by criteria that have little to do with medical knowledge and expertise—personality, appearance, what a friend at work said.

A more objective criterion is whether the physician is board certified. To be board certified in any field or specialty, a physician must pass a specific national examination in that field. Certification is overseen by national boards and the exam may include practical as well as written components. Some medical practices and hospitals *require* board certification, which is more common today than ever before.

You can also look up physicians on *healthgrades.com*. This site includes information about the doctor's training, board certification, malpractice history, and specialties. It includes personal accounts by patients about their experiences. It's a little jarring to see doctors rated in the fashion of burger joints and carpet cleaners, but the commentary on MDs I am familiar with has been spot on.

Medical Doctors and Osteopaths

When most people think of physicians, they conjure up traditional medical doctors (MDs or allopaths), who comprise about ninety percent of the field. Doctors of osteopathy (DOs) make up the rest, and osteopathy is growing quickly. About a quarter of all new medical students are in osteopathic programs, and osteopaths are expected to make up twenty percent of the medical field by 2030.

So, what's the difference? Both require four years of medical school, three years of post-graduate residency, and state licensing. Much of the distinction involves an osteopathic philosophical approach that is more holistic, regarding the entire body and its systems as interrelated, with a greater emphasis on musculoskeletal manipulation.

In general, you'll do just fine with either for primary care or family medicine.

Medical Specialists

Most American medical care in the twenty-first century begins with the primary care physician (PCP) or family medicine practitioner. When your medical problems veer into particular organ systems, however, medical care can move in all sorts of different directions.

Cardiologists, dermatologists, orthopedists, podiatrists, pediatricians, gastroenterologists, urologists, gynecologists, oncologists, neurologists, ophthalmologists—this incomplete list goes on and on, followed closely by a wide array of surgical specialists.

Medical specialties have become increasingly obscure and even a specialist may deal with a very narrow range of problems. You may also discover that your particular medical problem calls for a sub-specialist. An epileptologist, for instance, is a neurologist who focuses on epileptic seizures.

In the current American medical world, your access to these specialists is likely to be determined by your private insurance policy or your Medicare or Medicaid coverage. It's important to determine from the beginning whether a recommended specialist is covered within your network to avoid later financial surprises. It's also usually necessary to get approval from your insurance to consult one at all.

Sometimes, however, advance research isn't possible.

When you're riding an ER-bound ambulance with lights and sirens, and require emergency surgery, time is not a luxury you can afford. Nor can you just ask the doctor, since a staggering number of physicians have no personal knowledge of where their services fit into different payment systems.

Everybody hopes for the best and figures they'll sort it out later. Eventually they do, though the endings can be decidedly unhappy and have been known to involve bankruptcy.

Doctors in the Hospital

In the previous century, the doctor you'd see while in the hospital would be the same one you'd see before and after you were hospitalized. No more.

Emergency room doctors take care of whoever comes into the emergency room at any time, with any problem. This may be as straightforward as x-raying and wrapping a sprained ankle or as complex as ordering immediate clot-busting treatment for a stroke. Diagnosis is central to their work.

ER doctors do not treat patients outside of the emergency room and do not follow up after initial treatment, diagnosis, referral to other medical personnel, or hospital admission. Once you leave the ER in any direction, you won't see that ER doctor again unless you revisit the emergency room.

Hospitalists are licensed physicians who oversee the care of patients within the hospital. They may also have medical specialties with outside practices. Like the ER docs, they handle whoever comes through the door, from admission until the wheelchair ride out the front door to go home.

Intensivists are hospitalists who work only in intensive care or cardiac care.

Physician Assistants and Nurse Practitioners
Physician assistants (PAs) and **nurse practitioners** (NPs) are two relatively new occupations positioned on a tier between doctors and nurses. Both work in close association with physicians and perform many of the same functions.

These can include physical exams, diagnosis and treatment of illness, ordering and interpreting lab tests, assisting in some surgeries, writing prescriptions, and making rounds in rehab facilities and hospitals. In an increasing number of medical practices, they handle more routine issues to free up the doctor's time for more complicated cases.

Physician assistants have at least two years of college, rigorous and specialized training, and licenses to practice issued by their home states. Nurse practitioners are registered nurses with advanced training and are also state licensed.

The care you receive from either is likely to be excellent.

PAs and NPs are often scheduled for longer patient appointments than doctors, giving them more time to answer questions, explain things clearly, and follow up where necessary. In long-term caregiving situations that are relatively stable, you may find yourself working with them on a routine basis and consulting with the physician less frequently.

Because both come out of training pathways other than medical school, there's an added bonus: they often have much better people skills than the physicians they are associated with.

Nurses and Technicians

Nurses and technicians are discussed together here because there tends to be a lot of overlap on who does what, both from one facility to the next and from one location to the next. In general, the larger the hospital or facility, the more likely it is to have very specifically trained personnel. Six different technical specialists at a metropolitan teaching hospital might cover the functions handled by one cross-trained tech at a rural hospital in Wyoming.

You will encounter all the occupations listed below in most hospitals. Doctors' offices are more likely to have LPNs or LVNs as assistants.

Registered nurses (RNs) have completed an associate degree in nursing or a hospital-based training program and passed the national nursing license exam. Many have BS degrees as well.

Licensed practical nurses (LPNs) have completed a training program and passed a national licensing exam. In Texas and California, they are known as **licensed vocational nurses** (LVNs).

Certified nurse's aides (CNAs) are more involved in personal care than medical treatment.

Medical technicians don't come into contact with patients as often and many work entirely behind the scenes. They manage most of the imaging equipment as well as lab procedures and treatment administration.

Paramedics are **emergency medical technicians** (EMTs) who specialize in emergency stabilization and transport.

Therapists

The first thing many people think of when they hear the word "therapist" is psychotherapy, either from a psychiatrist (a licensed MD with advanced training) or a psychologist, who is not a physician but has specialized training in mental illness and interpersonal relations and is also licensed.

If your loved one is dealing with a mental health situation as either a primary or secondary medical problem, you will definitely want this type of help. Serious illness also often results in depression, which is hardly surprising and may lead to a mental health consultation.

Antidepressants are often prescribed by primary care physicians and specialists handling major medical problems. To avoid bad interactions, it's extremely important that everybody on the medical team has access to the patient's current medications list (*see* CHAPTER FOUR: DIAGNOSIS, TREATMENT, AND MEDICATION).

The patient may refuse to see a psychotherapist or to cooperate if the session is thrust upon them. Unfortunately, there isn't much you can do about that beyond being persuasive with your loved one as best you know how.

The caregiver may also suffer from depression, for obvious reasons. It's hard to see someone you love suffer in any fashion. If they are facing difficult treatment and/or a difficult prognosis, it's a hundred times worse.

There is no dishonor in bringing this up with your own PCP, who may have specific suggestions—pharmaceutical or otherwise—or refer you to a mental health specialist.

If you or the patient is referred, *go.*

Physical therapists (PTs) are commonly involved in caregiving situations, most often to help somebody regain previous capabilities after an accident, surgery, or any kind of severe and debilitating medical crisis.

Accidents of any sort involving broken bones are almost certain to require some physical therapy. This may be handled in the doctor's office or be referred to a dedicated therapy facility.

If hospitalization is involved for orthopedic surgery, PT will usually start in the hospital. It may then progress to an inpatient rehab facility, especially if the patient is older or lives alone, and will certainly include follow-up both at a PT facility and with home exercises.

Joint replacements have become almost as commonplace as tonsillectomies once were. Most joint replacements are voluntary. In this case, PT helps the body adjust to once again having a functional knee or hip or other joint. Usually that adjustment is relatively easy but does require oversight.

Physical therapy may also be recommended for patients recovering from brain events such as strokes, aneurysms, tumors, and traumatic brain injuries. Here the brain *and* various body parts must be retrained to work together to perform functions that they used to handle automatically.

Because of the complexities of interacting with a damaged brain, this kind of PT may take a long time, with results that are less than ideal.

Occupational therapists (OTs) live in the world of adaptation. That adaptation may involve learning or relearning skills as basic as how to button your shirt or hold a spoon. Occupational therapists can also provide guidance on reconfiguring a living space to accommodate new physical realities—everything from building a wheelchair ramp to relocating frequently-used items more conveniently.

Occupational therapists may work out of an office or facility. Some will visit the home either for assessment or to continue OT exercises. Brain-related OT may take a long time and a huge amount of homework, day after day, to make significant progress.

Speech therapists (STs) do exactly what their name suggests. They work to improve vocal communication for children with speech delays or difficulties, and for adults recovering from medical problems that have damaged or impaired talking or swallowing.

This therapy may begin in a rehab facility but will almost certainly be continued in the therapist's office. As with many types of occupational therapy, a great deal of practice and repetition may be necessary to regain lost abilities.

The Dress Code

In the recent past, doctors wore white lab coats with their names stitched above the pocket and nurses wore crisp white dresses, white nylons with sensible white shoes, and distinctive starched caps representing their nursing schools.

Today's medical dress code is a lot more relaxed but also more complicated. In this more complex world, you aren't likely to automatically recognize *anybody* by what they're wearing, though many doctors still wear white lab coats.

Scrubs are the medical wardrobe baseline and some institutions have all their staff wear the same style and color, which only makes matters more confusing. You'll need to learn to read and interpret name badges. If you're dealing with more than one medical group or facility, you may need to figure out player identification techniques and themes for each of them.

If you're confused about who's who, politely ask who you are dealing with and why. "Forgive me, but I'm a little confused" is an excellent way to begin, and far better than "Who on earth are *you?*"

Telemedicine

Telemedicine, also known as telehealth, limped along for years with little use or attention.

Many health care providers already offered such online communications as email appointment reminders and prescription renewal requests. Others permitted patients to view test results and other medical info on a personal medical portal. A few setups allowed nurse-practitioners in remote clinics to communicate with supervising physicians via imaging technology, with or without the patient as Exhibit A. Some VA hospitals were experimenting with telecommunication to monitor ongoing treatment or conditions such as hypertension.

Isolated parts of the country can be far removed from significant (or any) medical facilities and personnel. On the opposite extreme, transportation to and from routine medical monitoring in major metropolitan areas can be difficult, time-consuming, and expensive.

Implementation of telemedicine seemed a useful solution to both problems, but most health insurance providers refused to cover such consultations.

Then came the COVID-19 pandemic.

The nation's day-to-day medical services made big changes, pretty much overnight. People were being urged or ordered to stay at home. A significant number of older physicians fell into a high-risk age category that made in-person interactions with patients dangerous and inadvisable.

Elective surgeries and non-urgent consultations could be postponed, but people continued to have other health problems.

Doctors needed to learn quickly how to manage technology that would allow them to examine, diagnose, and treat patients at a distance. An impressive number rose to the occasion.

Simultaneously, health insurance providers, including Medicare, began to cover this kind of medical service.

Moving forward beyond the pandemic, some of these changes are likely to remain. The reality is that they proved effective and efficient for a lot of medical situations.

Arguably none of these situations are as ideal as sitting in the same room with a physician who is engaged and concerned about your health.

But telemedicine is the future.

MEDICAL FACILITIES

Hospitals

Not all hospitals are created equal.

There are about six thousand hospitals in the United States that meet the registration requirements of the American Hospital

Association (AHA), though not all are AHA members. About a quarter of hospitals are investor-owned, for-profit institutions. Another quarter are operated by various government entities and the remaining half are non-government, not-for-profit community hospitals.

Non-profit, in the case of hospitals, does not mean that there isn't plenty of money being charged to patients and whatever carriers insure them.

General or **community hospitals** can be any size, often depending on location. They treat medical and surgical patients and generally have an emergency room, laboratories, and intensive care unit (ICU).

Teaching hospitals are affiliates of medical schools, universities, and nursing schools. Physicians at teaching hospitals may specialize in very narrow or obscure research areas. Med students and residents working under their supervision may be more involved in actual care.

Specialty hospitals focus on one particular type of disease or medical treatment. They include hospitals for children, childbirth, geriatric care, psychiatric patients, and trauma victims.

Clinics and **surgery centers** are geared toward treatment that does not require overnight stays. Some are government-operated, but increasingly they are owned and operated by private medical personnel or partnerships.

Hospitals of all sorts are ranked and graded by various organizations and magazines, generally based on their areas of specialty. *Healthgrades.com* has its own ratings system and is useful for learning more about the hospitals in your area.

Hospital-Acquired Infections

A very disturbing element of twenty-first century hospital care is the prevalence and severity of infections acquired by patients while they are hospitalized.

These are mean and nasty bacteria and viruses and they love hanging out around already-weakened potential hosts. These bugs are experts at hitchhiking on mobile equipment or slipping into rooms with food delivery carts or jumping off traveling blood pressure monitors.

You want to do everything possible to avoid having your loved one attacked by these infections, which can cause long-lasting or permanent problems if they don't kill you outright. Antibiotics can help, of course, but bacterial hospital infections are increasingly resistant to even the strongest ones, and antibiotics are useless against viral infections.

Pneumonia is the most common infection and frequently shows up in patients in the ICU or on ventilators. It also is often contracted by patients in skilled nursing facilities.

MRSA (methicillin-resistant *Staphylococcus aureus*) tends to start on the skin and spreads very quickly. If caught and treated fast, these infections respond to antibiotics, but when left to themselves, they can lead to sepsis (blood poisoning) and death.

Clostridium difficile is nowhere as cute as its nickname, C. diff. This intestinal infection often results from major treatment by strong antibiotics, which wipe out the protective probiotics that normally live in a patient's digestive tract. It is notoriously difficult to cure and can return repeatedly after the patient is discharged.

How can you tell if your loved one is being attacked by one of these opportunistic predators? You are the best possible observer because you know the patient so well. Watch for rapid or serious changes in condition, including fever, rapid heartbeat and/or breathing, rashes, and confusion.

If you see these developments, tell the attending nurses and doctors immediately, and make enough of a fuss to be sure that your concerns are addressed right away. Every minute of delay can be dangerous. Or deadly.

Protect the Patient

Yes, protecting patients *is* supposed to be the hospital's job, and the people involved in your loved one's care are just as eager as you are to get them home safely, ASAP. At the same time, staff is usually limited and often overextended.

You can make a real difference just by paying close attention to absolutely everything.

Stay informed and make notes.

Know what treatments are in progress, which are expected, and when they all occur. You may not understand the equipment your loved one is hooked up to, but you can make sure it's still plugged in after the cleaning staff leaves. If there's a new machine, ask what it is and what it does. Mark surgical sites with black marker so nobody starts to replace the wrong knee.

Get to know the day-to-day staff who care for the patient, and **be nice to everybody**, even if you don't like them or are concerned that they aren't paying enough attention.

Even a forced smile can make a big difference. Learn names if you can and use them. If you don't already know the doctors, particularly hospitalists and new specialists, find out when they usually come in for rounds and be there when they're likely to show up. Have questions written down and ready.

Humanize the patient, particularly if they are unconscious or exceptionally cranky. Pictures on the bedside table are an easy way to do this, reminding everyone that in healthier days, the patient is happy and cheerful and beloved by family and friends. (If the patient is always a cantankerous jerk, you can probably still find pictures that suggest otherwise.)

We all learned the importance of keeping things clean during the COVID-19 pandemic. You should assume that you can do a better job for your own special patient than the folks who are also responsible for the rest of the building.

In any new room, wipe everything down with antibacterial wipes and pay particular attention to the tray table, bedside rails, call buttons, and every part of the bathroom. Door handles, light switches, curtain pulls, and the visitor's chair are likely to be loaded with germs.

Keep your personal stuff out of the room, including the purse or backpack you normally set down wherever you happen to be. Don't eat the patient's food or bring in food, and **do not use the patient's bathroom under any circumstances.**

Bring in a giant bottle of hand sanitizer and offer it to every person who enters the room with a big smile.

Repeat all of this daily. Or more often.

Skilled Nursing Facilities AKA Nursing Homes

Whatever they're called, these places are designed for recovering patients not yet ready to go home after hospitalization, or those with ongoing health problems that make it impossible to care for them at home. Nearly all of these patients are older.

Those recovering from surgery, including joint replacements, tend to recover uneventfully and go home greatly improved. Patients not necessarily on a road to improved health may be unconscious or comatose.

Memory care facilities for dementia patients are more specialized and offer safeguards against difficult behaviors, starting with exit doors that can't be operated by the patient. Memory care patients often come directly out of household environments. An effort is usually made to create a homey atmosphere, including group dining and accessible but confined outdoor areas.

There's no need to dwell on the terrible things that can and do happen in the worst of nursing homes. A short list includes neglect, restraints, incompetence, theft, and bedsores—in an environment that smells unpleasant and isn't particularly clean.

Insurance of any sort—employer-based, individual, or governmental through Medicare and/or Medicaid—at best covers only a limited stay, usually immediately after hospital discharge. Pay close attention to those limits because skilled nursing is quite expensive. Even those with long-term care insurance often have unpleasant surprises.

Costs vary significantly according to location. A median-priced private room in least-expensive Oklahoma costs over $60,000 a year, skyrocketing to over $275,000 for the same room in Alaska. Most locations offer a wide range of services and costs, but finding the right place for your loved one can be frustrating and time-consuming. And you need to do it in person.

If the hospital has a social worker, that person can help you through this transition period.

Also, whether or not you live nearby, you may want to hire a geriatric case manager to help you negotiate this process. These people are familiar with the local options and can steer you in the right direction for your loved one and your budget.

If you don't live nearby, a geriatric case manager can also be your eyes on the ground, making regular but unscheduled visits to check up.

With skilled nursing or memory care, you need to pay attention to everything and everybody. That's easy enough in the short run, but much more difficult over time, especially if the patient is difficult or unresponsive.

You should definitely get to know the staff and cultivate relationships with them with simple gifts of grocery-store flowers or candy. Ask questions. Smile.

And don't beat yourself up if the situation isn't perfect. All you can do is your best.

FOUR
DIAGNOSIS, TREATMENT, AND MEDICATION

Nearly all caregiving requires diagnosis and some kind of treatment plan. Most also involve medication. All operate in what is intended to be a symbiotic relationship.

For some patients, they may be quite simple. Others involve a breathtaking combination of all sorts of things. Many may be new to you and also new to your health care team. The medical world changes daily, often for the better.

DIAGNOSIS AND TREATMENT

Diagnosis and treatment are often so interrelated in major caregiving situations that it isn't possible to separate them.

By the time a patient gets a firm diagnosis for any medical problem, there may have been weeks or months of testing and lab work and drug experimentation to determine exactly what is happening. This may involve specialists upon specialists, some of whom flatly contradict one another. It can be both a challenge and a mess.

A central concern is that without knowing exactly what a misbehaving body is doing, some possible treatments may make things even worse. This can be true even with the best intentions, a highly informed patient, and an excellent physician. Stuff happens.

With an accident or an obvious physical crisis, treatment almost always begins before an official diagnosis.

Electronic Diagnosis

Electronic tools are being designed to assist in diagnosis by keeping all possible answers to a medical question open until there is reason to eliminate them.

One reason for this is obvious. Medical personnel often reach a tentative diagnosis based on reported symptoms very early, sometimes before even seeing the patient. Having done so, they may proceed to the customary treatment for that problem without fully exploring other possible diagnoses. A doctor who recognizes a specific list of symptoms associated with Whosi-whatitis may conclude that's the problem without further investigation, when in fact the patient has Similaritis, which requires entirely different treatment.

Occasionally something that quacks like a duck is actually a nightingale with a sore throat. Everybody's heard about the patient sent home with routine instructions for treating a stomachache or headache or cold, when the problem turned out to be something else altogether.

The growing field of electronic diagnosis is based on a series of checklists. A computer (which can be accessed online from anywhere) takes the list of symptoms and checks their entire range of possibilities. Examination and patient questioning will eliminate some of these possibilities and add others. The computer can then factor in this additional data to give the doctor or other health technician a more complete diagnostic picture.

Most of this kind of diagnosis is in its infancy, but it's the wave of the future.

Second Opinions

Second opinions are not an insult to doctors, and many insurance companies insist on them before performing certain surgeries or procedures. This may help alleviate or avoid the kind of medical tunnel vision that can result from a speedy or inaccurate diagnosis. It can also provide reassurance.

You may need to pay out of pocket for a second opinion, but this is money well spent if you are uncertain or uncomfortable with what you've been told, or with a proposed treatment plan.

Making Decisions

Sometimes decisions are made for you. By the time choice comes into play, a patient may be well down their own medical highway and perhaps lucky to still be alive.

Accidents are the most common example of this. Heart attacks and strokes are another. All share the elements of uncertainty and surprise.

One minute everything is sailing along just as it always does and then—*Bam!!!*—everything changes. Those at the epicenter of such events must suddenly keep up with developments and notify family members and juggle responsibilities and ask that horrifying question: Now what?

There are always going to be *Now what?* moments in caregiving, but mostly they can be approached in a less frenzied manner that allows time for reflection, discussion, and research.

Either way, it needs to be clear who has the authority to make these decisions.

Advance directives are the single most important thing that anybody can do to assure that their wishes for treatment will be used by their medical team. This is a legal document that goes by various names in different states and will be discussed fully in CHAPTER FIVE: THE PAPER JUNGLE.

Advance directives name a person authorized to make medical decisions if the patient is unable to do so. They also designate what types of treatment the patient wishes in specific medical situations. Without legal paperwork in place, the spouse is first in line to make decisions, followed by children, parents, and siblings.

In advanced or deteriorating medical situations, more specific documents may apply. The most common is a DNR: do not resuscitate (*see* CHAPTER FIVE: THE PAPER JUNGLE).

All of these legal documents are state-specific, so you need to be sure that you are using the correct form for the patient's state of residence.

Matters can get really messy if the patient is unconscious, semi-conscious, or if the illness or accident involves brain damage.

Decision-making has the potential to get ugly. Make every effort to work together as a family and respect the patient's wishes, even if they are not what you personally might do. De-escalate as much as possible when there are conflicting opinions. The last thing you want is to end up in court, fighting with the people who should be supporting both the caregiver and the patient.

If you're really at loggerheads, try to find an impartial mediator (either inside or outside the family) who is respected by everyone. A religious professional can be very helpful if everyone is part of the same faith community.

Imaging

Diagnostic imaging used to be limited to an x-ray machine and a lead apron. The imaging discussed here is separate and distinct from the radiation treatment used for cancer.

X-rays remain the core of the diagnostic imaging family, using electromagnetic radiation to provide interior photographs of the body. X-rays are digital now, offering greater immediacy than the bulky life-sized films of the past, which required chemical processing and special storage.

The result is the same, however: a black-and-white picture with a sharp contrast between soft and hard tissues. Dental and orthopedic x-rays can provide definitive diagnoses, but other uses may be less certain. Preliminary x-rays may indicate an unexpected mass or tumor that can be further explored with a more sophisticated or focused type of imaging. The most familiar instance of this is mammography followed up by ultrasound.

Ultrasound uses sonography to create images of soft tissue by mapping sound waves as they pass through the body. Fetal images posted online to announce pregnancies are ultrasounds, as are later pregnancy images that may reveal gender.

Ultrasound can be used to determine how a soft-tissue body process is functioning or to identify stones in a kidney or gall bladder. To position organs for better imaging, patients are sometimes told to drink vast quantities of water and fill the bladder. This moves everything else around.

CT scans, also known as **CAT scans**, allow the radiologist to look at image slices of an organ or part of the body to see where abnormalities might be tucked away. If you were making a CT scan of an orange, the process would reveal the number and location of seeds. CT imagery often also uses radio contrast agents such as iodine, injected to offer sharper contrast. The machinery is large and whirs as it rotates around the patient's body.

MRI scans are magnetic resonance images and can offer better contrast resolution than CT, without using ionizing radiation. MRIs are not popular among patients because they are noisy, may take a long time, and confine the patient in a tightly enclosed area. Open MRI equipment has been developed but is not yet readily available. Claustrophobic patients may require earplugs and mild sedation.

PET scans are positron emission tomography and are used almost exclusively to locate cancer metastases. PET scans create a multi-colored, 3-D view of the body to either track down an unidentified primary tumor or to identify locations where a cancer has spread or metastasized.

X-rays and ultrasounds are far more readily available and reasonably priced than CT, MRI, or PET scans, all of which require large and complex equipment. Portable CT scanning is sometimes used in hospital or office settings.

Surgery

Being able to get inside the human body to fix things is a relatively recent development in medical history.

Body parts can now be replaced as well as removed or patched up. Wounds and scars are often much smaller and recovery faster and easier. Lengthy post-op hospital stays have been shortened or even eliminated. The patient shows up at sunrise and is back home by sunset.

A hospital may not even be involved. Freestanding surgery centers handle all sorts of operations and are often owned by the surgeons themselves.

Laparoscopy is a minimally invasive form of surgery that substitutes tiny "keyhole" incisions for larger old-style abdominal openings. Carbon dioxide is pumped in between the skin and organs. Instruments are passed through the keyhole incisions to perform necessary tasks. Tiny cameras show the operating field inside this impromptu balloon.

Laparoscopic surgery lacks the advantage of touch and palpation common to previous abdominal surgeries, but it's not as hard on the body and recovery is usually faster.

Robotic surgery is increasingly used in brain and prostate surgeries, with the potential to move into other areas. It is useful in situations where precision is crucial and accessibility limited. The actual operation is conducted by machinery rather than hands. Younger surgeons who grew up on computer gaming are today's robotic surgery specialists.

Diagnostic surgery is less common than it used to be because of improved imaging techniques, but it still comes into play where a biopsy (direct tissue examination in a lab) is the only way to accurately determine the nature of a tumor. Most diagnostic surgeries are cancer-related.

Inoperable tumors are located in difficult-to-access places, usually in close proximity to other vital organs likely to be damaged by attempted removal of the tumor. Debulking such tumors as much as possible without harming other healthy nearby tissues sets up a balancing act that can buy time.

Orthopedic surgery treats the musculoskeletal system, including bones, joints, ligaments, tendons, muscles, and nerves. It may be either elective or emergency. Elective operations are used to fix or improve problems that are either congenital, continuations of previous bone repairs, or the result of friction, sports, and/or age.

Emergency orthopedic surgeries arise out of falls and other accidents and are much more prevalent in older people with brittle bones. Women with osteoporosis are at particular risk.

Joint replacements are a growing field and the number of joints now available continues to grow. Lifelong athletes need them, but so do lifelong couch potatoes. Devices are made of ceramic, plastic, and/or metal. Technically these are elective operations that people often regret putting off as long as they did.

Cancer Treatment

Cancer treatment requires special attention because it is both ubiquitous and individualized.

Why is there so much cancer?

Plenty of theories range from genetics to environmental pollution to exposure to bad things at home or at work—to a lot of cockamamie theories that bear little relation to reality. Almost everybody facing cancer grapples at some point with the *Why?* question, but try to let it go as soon as you possibly can.

This is a good place to remind you that people are going to want to share their personal or secondhand or multiple hearsay cancer stories with you whether you want to hear them or not. You may need to be forceful or even rude in order to shut somebody up.

The appropriate response: *I just can't talk about this right now. Keep us in your thoughts and prayers.* Feel free to cry at this point, and you may not need to fake it. Then walk away if you possibly can.

Cancer isn't actually one disease at all, but an entire family of afflictions linked by uncontrolled cell growth in organs. Not all tumors are cancer, but any new or unusual lumps should definitely be checked by a physician. A non-cancerous tumor is considered to be benign.

Some cancers exist as aberrations in blood or lymphatic fluids, with no tumor at all.

Cancer treatments share common ground. You can learn much more about the current available regimens for your loved one's type of cancer from the American Cancer Society website, *cancer.org*.

One thing most of these treatments share is that you are subjecting the human body to what would otherwise be considered serious abuse. Chemotherapy voluntarily puts poisons into the body. Radiation zaps patients over and over again. Immunotherapy may involve a dangerous infection of some other sort.

These treatments can be very, very nasty. They can also work miracles.

Cancer also has a language all its own.

Stages of cancer are usually numbered 1–4 and refer to how advanced the particular cancer is, with stage four being the worst.

Metastasis is when a cancer that began in one organ travels to afflict another unrelated one via the blood or lymph systems. Some cancers are discovered out of order, with the original tumor not immediately known and the metastasized one revealing itself first.

Oncologists are cancer treatment specialists and you will almost certainly be working with one. Most cancer treatments use a combination of surgery, radiation, and chemotherapy.

Side effects of different treatments can sometimes be far worse than the overt symptoms of the disease. Take them seriously and talk to the oncologist if the side effects seem out of line from what you were told to expect.

Surgery is often used to remove the tumor or as much of it as possible given its nature and location. Sometimes surgery will be delayed until after other treatments that are designed to reduce it in size. Surgical biopsy of affected tissue can provide a definitive diagnosis in uncertain cases.

Radiation is generally used repeatedly over a period of time to burn away tumor cells with highly targeted electromagnetic rays. Many radiation regimens require repetition five days a week for weeks or months on end. Weekends are free for recuperation, and never long enough.

The area in question may be tattooed, and specially constructed personal braces assure that exactly the same radiation pattern is followed every single time.

Radiation therapy is very hard on the body and generally exhausting. The exhaustion may dissipate over time but that isn't guaranteed. Appetite often fades away and radiation patients frequently lose a lot of weight.

Chemotherapy or chemo is what most people think of when you mention cancer treatment. It involves many different types of chemicals in various combinations. What they have in common is that they would normally be considered poisonous.

Chemo regimens vary greatly and your oncologist will work with you to fine-tune them as necessary. Chemo is likely to go on at intervals over a prolonged period—sometimes more than a year—and may involve anything from daily pills to monthly infusions.

A lot of chemotherapy is nauseating, so keep a bucket in the car.

Marijuana (cannabis) has a well-deserved reputation for alleviating that nausea and is now widely available in many forms that do not require inhaling smoke.

Many forms of chemo result in **hair loss**, which can be devastating—whether it is gradual or happens all at once in horrifying clumps. Hair lost to chemo usually does grow back, though it may not look or feel the same as what was lost during treatment. Insurance may cover wigs and there are all kinds of head coverings available.

It's still awful.

Chemo brain refers to a type of mental fuzziness that goes along with many types of cancer treatment, particularly for cancers of the female reproductive system. People joke about chemo brain, but it can be very real and very terrifying. The good news is that it usually improves with time.

Immunotherapy as cancer treatment is still in its early stages but holds great promise. This type of treatment uses a person's own immune system as a weapon against targeted cancer. The body tends not to reject cancerous tumors the way it might fight other sorts of disease intruders. Immunotherapy works to short-circuit those boundaries and let other types of infection attack the tumor.

Clinical trials are often available for cancer patients because there is so much cancer research that needs to be tested. They are usually available only as a last resort after all traditional treatments have been tried without success.

Autoimmune Disorders

Autoimmune disorders are very sneaky, complicated, and diffi-cult to diagnose.

The human body has an immune system designed to protect it from infections or infestations, but sometimes that system gets out of whack. Then the body mistakenly attacks itself under a wide range of different circumstances.

In some cases, the body works too hard to defend itself and in others it doesn't work hard enough. Either can cause an array of problems, and they make matters even more complex in major health crises. Sometimes they *create* those crises.

Familiar autoimmune diseases include lupus, Crohn's and IBD, alopecia, celiac disease, rheumatoid arthritis, multiple scle-rosis, type 1 diabetes, and psoriasis. Altogether there are about eighty of them and they are usually treated by specialists in the organ system under attack.

Whether or not your loved one's autoimmune disorder is di-rectly related to the health issue at hand, you'll want to coordinate with the specialist who is treating it to be sure that all treatments and therapies will be as compatible as possible with the disorder.

Mental Illness

Mental illness is wide ranging and highly individualized, both from person to person and from day to day.

Three bipolar patients, for example, may have widely differ-ent manifestations but all fit the diagnostic profile. They may or may not respond to any number of medications and therapies. And all of this has the potential to change over time, often dramatically.

That assumes that the patient stays on the meds, an assumption you can't always make. That also assumes that the mental illness hasn't informed the patient that there really isn't anything wrong, which can also happen. And that the patient isn't self-medicating with alcohol, marijuana, or illegal drugs.

If you are working with somebody with a history of mental illness, you are probably already familiar with at least the basics of their personal situation. If the caregiving problem has arisen from another type of illness or an accident, the mental health problems (and their current treatment) need to be factored in at every level.

It can be awkward to ask for help from both family members and outsiders in these cases. In part, the age-old stigma lingers. Also, everybody has opinions and viewpoints that may not correspond to the immediate situation. *Just snap out of it* has a very poor track record.

The patient should be working with a psychologist or psychiatrist or both. A psychiatrist is a medical doctor with specialized psychiatric training. A psychologist is not an MD but may also have a doctorate. Psychologists cannot prescribe drugs but usually work in conjunction with a psychiatrist when meds are advisable.

Talk therapy can be useful for some patients and worthless for others.

Medication is available in many categories: antidepressants, stimulants, antipsychotics, mood stabilizers, anxiolytics, depressants, and psychedelics. Finding the appropriate meds can be frustrating and time-consuming, and even when you find the golden combination and dosage, it may become ineffective over time.

Homeopathic medications should not be used in conjunction with prescribed medications.

There are all kinds of support groups for various types of mental illness and for the loved ones of the mentally ill. Look for one that addresses the specifics of your loved one's disease.

The best general source of information on all elements of all mental illness is the National Alliance on Mental Illness (NAMI), *nami.org*. You can start by downloading their free publication, *Circle of Care: A Guidebook for Mental Health Caregivers*.

Alzheimer's and Dementia

At the current rate of diagnosis, Alzheimer's and other forms of dementia will affect one out of every three American adults in their final years.

That's a scary number, particularly since people are living a good deal longer, and a lot of baby boomers made a fetish out of taking good care of themselves so their bodies would perform well for a very long time.

All Alzheimer's is dementia, but not all dementia is Alzheimer's. The reality is that it doesn't make a lot of difference.

There's little to say about dementia treatments, because at the moment there really aren't any. The best that most medical therapies can do is slightly delay additional deterioration. That's great, of course, but nowhere near an effective cure. The Food and Drug Administration (FDA) has recently approved the use of Aduhelm (aducanumab) as a monthly infusion to slow cognitive decline. The FDA is also requiring additional clinical trials because of uncertainty about the drug's effectiveness.

When other medication is prescribed, it's generally aimed at modulating mental health issues such as depression, anxiety, or anti-social behaviors. The caregiver needs to control the meds because the patient may not be able to keep track.

Almost everything involved in caring for somebody with dementia requires environmental modifications for your loved one's safety (*see* CHAPTER EIGHT: THE NEW NORMAL). Additional caregiving and housekeeping help are often needed. It is really, really hard for one caregiver to provide all the help and attention and patience that one dementia patient requires. Plus fix dinner and run the vacuum.

The good news, limited though it may be, is that excellent support and information is available through the Alzheimer's Association, *alz.org*.

Substance Abuse

Substance abuse is another matter altogether.

If you are caring for somebody with substance abuse problems in addition to other medical issues, it's important to understand that this can directly affect treatment for the medical issue. The doctor needs to know if the patient is putting away a bottle of wine every night on top of a handful of prescription drugs.

Addictions of all sorts can be mentally crippling and physically debilitating. In addition, there is the issue of *use* versus *abuse*. Some people are able to try almost anything without worrying about addiction, while others cannot take a single drink or smoke a single cigarette. Again, much of this is a matter of how the patient is hardwired.

People with substance abuse problems may be reluctant to seek help and highly resistant to attempts by others to guide them in that direction.

The most useful question in many substance situations is whether it is interfering with other aspects of the person's life. If so, then some kind of intervention may be necessary. Inpatient rehab may also be required to break addictive patterns under round-the-clock supervision.

Twelve-step programs such as Alcoholics Anonymous can be invaluable, and hotlines answer phone calls 24/7 from the anxious or desperate. Over 200 specialized programs exist for various forms of addiction, as well as such support groups for secondary victims such as Alanon, Alateen, and Adult Children of Alcoholics (ACA).

All are free and all take the concept of anonymity very seriously.

Alternative Treatments

Alternative treatments may involve holistic treatment, megavitamins and supplements, a special diet, massage therapy, acupuncture, acupressure, and all manner of special equipment.

In general, there's nothing wrong with any of this, and many healthy people include these elements in their daily life. Whether to continue most of them during treatment for a specific medical problem is an individual decision, but it's important to balance them with the medical advice you are given.

Keep in mind that if the patient takes supplements or vitamins or anything else that comes in a little bottle from the health food store, *these are medications*. They may interact badly with—or even block—prescribed medications or supervised treatment regimens.

Make sure that your doctor knows about all of the things the patient has been taking, especially if they continue to do so.

Doctors tend not to be very keen on alternative treatments, and you may have to accept a lecture when providing information on what the patient is (or isn't) doing. But it's absolutely crucial to include these items on current medication lists and to make sure health providers are aware of them (*see* CHAPTER TWO: GETTING ORGANIZED).

Be wary of alternative treatments that head into snake oil territory. These usually come up when traditional treatment isn't going as well as had been hoped. They often enter into a caregiving situation via one person, sometimes the patient.

Doctors *really* hate these.

Extremely unorthodox treatments deserve and require plenty of research because of the potential to cause harm, either on their own or from delaying or replacing more conventional treatment.

Being on the internet doesn't make something true. Nor does having a glossy ad on late night television. Pay attention to who's making the claims, what exactly those claims are, and what credentials that person or website may have. If at all possible, convince the patient to try more conventional therapies first.

Steve Jobs didn't, and it did not go well for him.

Medical Tourism

Medical tourism is a lot less glamorous than it sounds.

It may mean traveling halfway around the world for a pricey procedure not covered by insurance or driving to Tijuana for a root canal. Frequently it refers to getting expensive medications at a lower price from Mexico or Canada, either in person or by mail order.

For surgery or unorthodox medical treatments, patient and caregiver both need to be comfortable with travel and willing to spend a prolonged period in an unfamiliar environment where everybody is speaking a language you don't know. You can't just replace a knee and then hop back on a plane.

Plan carefully if you decide to do this and be sure to get travel insurance.

Palliative Care

Palliative care focuses on making the patient comfortable. It can be used at any stage of treatment for any kind of illness or injury. It is a supplement to care required for treatment of the medical problem, not a substitute.

It asks the question: Does this person feel as good as possible right now? If the answer is "no," then it looks for ways to change that.

Palliative care is often associated with hospice, after a patient agrees to no longer use the medical system to fight whatever has been attacking their body (*see* CHAPTER NINE: END OF LIFE ISSUES).

In the context of hospice, the goal is to make the patient as comfortable and pain free as possible. This may involve entirely different types of drugs from those used for treatment, as well as heavy doses of painkillers.

But for day-to-day caregiving, palliative care is relatively simple and may be as easy as giving the patient a (doctor-approved) anti-inflammatory such as acetaminophen or ibuprofen for a headache. Or drawing a nice warm bubble bath.

Consider drawing another bubble bath for yourself when the patient goes back to bed. You've earned it.

MEDICATION

Medication is any type of natural or chemical non-food material used to help with symptoms, to treat problems, or to prevent illness from occurring in the first place. It can be as simple as an herbal tea or as complicated as multi-part chemotherapy. It may be used for a limited period or taken indefinitely.

In other words, drugs.

Many drugs require a prescription, but plenty don't, and many other substances also qualify as drugs. Vitamins and supplements. Tobacco, alcohol, and caffeine. Herbs in any configuration from snipped-off-the-bush to brewed into a tea or tincture. Endorphins from exercise. Recreational drugs, which may also have medicinal uses.

Some people are very self-righteous about not adulterating their bodies with drugs. If you are caring for somebody who wants to avoid drugs as much as possible, it can be useful to emphasize that many are used only for the short-term.

Use It or Lose It

Here's the most important part: The patient needs to actually take a medication or it can't work.

A lot of people slack off on preventative drugs, such as blood pressure or cholesterol medications that bring unseen functions into equally unseen normal ranges. When you can't actually see or feel a result, it can be tempting not to bother.

This temptation can literally kill.

Categories of Medication

Pharmaceuticals don't just happen. Lengthy and complicated research and many levels of clinical trials are required to bring a drug to market, and most drugs never get that far. For every drug that makes it to your local pharmacy, thousands fall along the wayside.

Brand name drugs are available from a single manufacturer, though many variants of the same drug may be available from many companies.

Patented drugs are newly developed and designated as such by the U.S. Patent and Trademark Office. Patenting can begin anywhere from early research until a drug hits the shelf, and lasts for twenty years.

Exclusive drugs are designated as such by the Food and Drug Administration (FDA), which gives a manufacturer up to seven years before others may copy the drug.

Not all drugs are patented or exclusive, and indeed some commercial medications available from Big Pharma have been used for millennia. Colchicine, for example, is derived from the bulb of the autumn crocus and was probably used to treat gout by Henry VIII and Benjamin Franklin, along with various mummies in Egyptian tombs.

Generic drugs are bioequivalent versions of once-patented drugs, identical in every respect but price. They have been tested and approved by the FDA and may include different inert ingredients from each other and the original brand-name medication, a potential issue for those with sensitivities to things like gluten.

About two-thirds of all drugs sold in the United States are generic. Many states, the Veterans Administration, and a lot of insurance companies require that generics be dispensed when they are available. Medicare does not, which costs the government a billion or so dollars every year.

Many people (and physicians!) don't believe that generic drugs are as effective as their branded relatives, but there's not much in the line of evidence for this notion.

Over-the-counter (OTC) drugs are available to anyone, and you can drop them in your shopping cart without consulting a doctor or a pharmacist. Sometimes these are preparations that have been around for a long time, such as aspirin, but this designation is also given to meds that were once branded and available only by prescription. They may go generic at the same time as they go OTC, but this does not necessarily mean they will be inexpensive.

Herbal and homeopathic medications are drugs and can interact with other medications just as badly as if they were produced by pharmaceutical companies.

One of the biggest problems with herbals and homeopathics is the lack of enforceable standards. Three bottles from different companies that claim to be the same thing may contain wildly different amounts of the alleged active ingredients. Sometimes they don't contain *any* of the wonder component.

Over-the-counter weight-loss medications are a particular crapshoot because they tend to offer miracle cures to people accustomed to battling weight gain unsuccessfully. They can do more damage than good, often with no way to know until it's too late.

Orphan drugs treat diseases and conditions that are rare or obscure, with few diagnosed patients. Their effectiveness is often discovered accidentally, as a side effect of a prescribed medication being used to treat something unrelated. The best way to learn about them is from a specialist in that obscure disease or an online support group for it.

Off-label use of prescription medication is legal but uncommon. Like orphan drugs, these pharmaceutical surprises usually occur accidentally. They can seem like miracle drugs, particularly in instances where more conventional therapies have not worked.

The best-known example is Minoxidil, a blood pressure medication that also stimulates hair growth. Balding men with hypertension taking this drug were surprised to notice hair returning to scalps that had grown shiny. Thus was born the Rogaine industry.

Antibiotics

Antibiotics are known as miracle drugs, and rightly so. The correct antibiotic aimed at a bacterial infection can stop it in its tracks, sometimes almost instantly.

There are limits, however.

Antibiotics are basically useless against viral infections of any sort, which is why the doctor won't automatically prescribe them when you have a cold. They can wipe out the friendly flora in your digestive system or vagina and create secondary problems, so it's a good idea to take a probiotic at the same time and protect those systems.

In addition, bacteria are sneaky little things, very adaptable to getting around antibiotics that used to routinely wipe them out. As a result, many conventional antibiotics are no longer effective against germs they used to fight successfully. And the heavy-duty antibiotics that have been developed as a result can wreak havoc on a patient's system. The most notable example is Clostridium difficile, or C. diff, a common hospital-acquired infection that arises after extensive use of antibiotics.

Antibiotics are sometimes prescribed to ward off secondary infections ready to join the party when a viral infection occurs. An antibiotic boost during a lingering viral infection may be just the assistance your body needs to wipe out opportunistic bugs so your body can heal.

It's important to finish the entire antibiotic prescription even if you start to feel better before the pills are gone. Check with the pharmacist or read the small print to find out when they should be taken relative to food. This allows the medication to work more effectively and can also avoid gastric distress.

If your loved one is reluctant to take antibiotics for any reason and you are convinced that they are being wisely and correctly prescribed, emphasize the positive.

These are miracle drugs.

Painkillers

Pain relief is a necessary part of the treatment for many diseases and conditions, and painkillers range from the relatively benign to the potentially deadly. The balance you want to strike is providing sufficient medication to counteract discomfort without zonking out the patient or setting up additional problems.

Over-the-counter pain meds will work for many people and many types of pain and should always be tried first. All are called **NSAIDs**, nonsteroidal anti-inflammatory drugs.

Acetylsalicylic acid (aspirin) used to be very popular but has fallen out of favor because it can promote bleeding and also because other, more effective OTC drugs are available. Aspirin is widely used in very small doses as a preventive against heart attacks.

Acetaminophen (Tylenol) is used for pain and fever relief. When taken at higher levels or for longer periods than recommended, it can cause permanent and sometimes deadly kidney and liver damage.

Ibuprofen (Advil, Motrin) and **Naproxen** (Aleve) are both widely used for day-to-day pain.

All of these are available in giant bottles at the big box store, which leads some folks to pop them like M&Ms. This is a really bad idea and can result in internal bleeding. If a patient has pain that isn't relieved after a reasonably short period, a physician should be consulted.

If the doctor recommends one over another, follow instructions because there's usually a good reason. All are available in generic versions at relatively low cost.

Narcotic pain relievers are another matter.

These are subject to abuse and can lead to addiction. America's opioid crisis has killed countless people, mostly young and otherwise healthy, and has focused much-needed attention on abuse not just by users but also by the pharmaceutical industry, which promoted them in sometimes shocking ways.

When you need narcotic painkillers, it's generally for a very serious reason and the relief they provide can be astonishing. Use them only as the physician recommends, but don't be afraid to take them when necessary.

Patients with a history of addiction and those who fear all painkillers should discuss these issues with the medical team. Common sense is a good arbiter here.

Medical Marijuana

Medical marijuana until very recently was limited to a handful of states and considered quite provocative.

Those days are over.

The legalization of medical marijuana, now commonly known as cannabis, began in California in 1996 and reached a tipping point around the time some states began to legalize the use of recreational marijuana. Now it's more unusual to find a state that doesn't permit it than one that does.

When legally available, it is generally sold through dispensaries. Knowledgeable budtenders can direct you to the most appropriate type of cannabis for your specific problem and the best way for a particular patient to administer it.

Not all cannabis is the same. Decades of clandestine horticultural experimentation and crossbreeding by outlaw botanists have produced a wide range of strains with an equally wide range of effects and benefits.

It is no longer necessary to roll a leafy substance into cigarette form or pack it into a pipe and smoke it. Cannabis still comes in that form, but it is also available in a wide range of edibles, concentrates, oils, tinctures, and creams designed to be more specific and user-friendly in a world turned firmly against the notion of smoking anything.

What can cannabis be used to treat?

The short answer is just about anything, but the evidence for this is almost exclusively anecdotal. Cannabis first gained grudging medical attention for combatting nausea in chemotherapy patients and was later employed by HIV/AIDS patients as an appetite stimulant. It is now widely used for pain relief, to relieve anxiety, as a sleep aid, and to combat all sorts of other symptoms, including rare forms of epilepsy in children.

Very little research exists about the medical use and effectiveness of cannabis for two important reasons.

First, it is classified by the Drug Enforcement Administration (DEA) as a Schedule I drug, along with heroin, LSD, and peyote. This is considered the worst possible type of drug, with no legitimate use. Second, the pathway to approval for research in the United States has been virtually nonexistent. The tiny number of scientists granted research permission have been required to use only governmental cannabis grown at a single location in Mississippi and generally regarded as inferior to ditch weed.

If you and your loved one think that medical marijuana might be a useful therapy, you will need a physician's approval in states that permit medical but not recreational marijuana. Not all doctors will agree to this, but if you call a dispensary, they can probably steer you toward somebody who will be more patient-friendly.

And if everything is illegal where you live, ask a young friend or relative for help. They are likely to know a lot more about this than you realize.

Side Effects and Interactions

When you insert an unfamiliar material into the body, there may be unintended side effects. This is equally true of expensive patented drugs and cheapo cough syrups, and you generally don't know there's going to be a problem until it happens.

Always take the pharmacist counseling offered with new medications. Doctors may mention common potential side effects, but don't count on it. You can also read the paperwork dispensed with some drugs, though you'll probably need a magnifying glass.

Common side effects may be digestive issues, headaches, weakness, sleepiness, sleeplessness, agitation, muscle aches, dizziness, confusion—in short, pretty much anything.

Other side effects may be much more serious, which is why all those glossy TV drug commercials have the familiar voiceover warnings about endless potential calamities, including death.

If the patient experiences serious side effects, you should always inform the physician promptly.

The best way to figure out if you're likely to have a drug interaction is to Google the name of the medication or supplement plus "interaction" with the other medication you are wondering about (or, even better, all other meds). You're likely to find some unsettling surprises.

If the patient is taking a lot of different medications prescribed by various physicians, along with a supplement or ten, pharmacists will usually evaluate them for you. Check first, then dump all the bottles into a bag and take them in.

Pharmacists know this stuff better than anyone. It's their job.

Keeping Track of Medications

Medication needs to be administered at the appropriate times and in the amounts prescribed. There are lots of ways to do this, starting with opening every bottle every time.

The easiest approach is to get a plastic dispenser with separate containers for seven days. These are available at any pharmacy and can come with as little as one row or as many as four rows for different times of the day. You fill these dispensers once a week and open the proper compartment at the proper time.

Note: you don't need to fill pill dispensers on Sunday if it's not convenient for you. Pick a day of the week and stick to it.

Fancier versions exist with bells and whistles, sometimes literally, to let you know it's time to take your meds and to dispense a previously loaded set of pills for that time.

Some pharmacies now offer a service that will package and label pills that are to be taken together at a particular time. Some also have apps that will read a label and give instructions out loud.

If the patient is confused or unable to manage filling and using any level container, that task automatically defaults to the caregiver.

The Cost of Drugs

Drugs cost too much.

Everybody seems to agree on this, and yet somehow the United States still spends more per capita on pharmaceuticals than any nation on earth, with costs rising regularly and usually without obvious reason.

The political background to this outrage has a lot to do with lobbying by the health care industry. Health care interests spend more on lobbying Congress than the defense industry does. Yes, really.

Health insurance usually provides partial or complete payment of medication costs, though this is only useful if you have health insurance. Even then, large deductibles and copays may put needed medication out of reach.

Medicare offers drug coverage as Part D, created in 2003 and paid for by the insured through affiliated insurance companies. Medicare is forbidden by Congress to negotiate with pharmaceutical companies to lower costs.

If you're on your own nickel for drug purchases, it pays to check the local and online options for the best price. These prices can vary substantially in the same town and even on the same block.

Shopping across the border helps some people keep drug costs down, whether they actually visit pharmacies in Mexico and Canada, or order online and hope for the best. The biggest problem here, apart from inaccessibility, is that there's no guarantee that what you purchase abroad is the actual medication and not a clever counterfeit.

Meanwhile, drug costs continue to soar.

The cost of insulin to treat diabetes, for example, has sky-rocketed. Insulin has tripled in price just since the turn of the twenty-first century, putting it out of financial reach for many patients. It's a tough call when the choice is dinner for the kids or a medication that will keep the breadwinner or one of those kids alive.

So, patients gamble and do without, or try to parcel out what they can afford by skipping doses or sharing a single prescription. These are all terrible solutions that can and do kill people.

Another common medication with a dramatic price rise is the asthma inhaler, which once had low-level, over-the-counter versions as well as inexpensive prescription ones. When the fluorocarbon propellants used to dispense the medicine were outlawed, Big Pharma seized the opportunity to jack up prices. Largely cosmetic changes, such as adding a meter to inhalers, allowed drug companies to eliminate generic versions and bump up all prices.

Identical asthma inhalers today cost three times as much in the United States as they do in Canada.

And what about new drugs?

If anything, the cost of new patented brand name medications is even more outrageous. This is commonly attributed to the costs of research and development, which can be quite high since most drugs never get past the R&D stage.

Single doses of chemotherapy drugs can cost tens of thousands of dollars. New miracle drugs advertised at great cost on television—the ones with happy users going about happy lives while the voiceover warns of side effects such as death—are priced so high that many drug companies offer programs to sell them cheaply to patients who couldn't otherwise afford them.

Pharmaceutical companies aggressively target physicians as well as potential consumers, though such overkill as paid vacations and expensive dinners are no longer common because the industry has actually regulated itself, at least a little. Information about perks and payments to doctors is technically available, though difficult to access. *ProPublica.org* has more information.

Meanwhile, if drug costs are overwhelming, be honest with your doctor. She may be able to provide some samples in the short run, or come up with another, less expensive option that will work just as well.

Drug Disposal

Do not flush drugs down the toilet.

Yes, everybody used to do it, and yes, it was a really easy way to get rid of the medication that didn't work or the leftover pills in an ancient bottle of OTC pain relievers.

The problem is that once these drugs become part of the wastewater system, they don't disappear, but merely dissolve. They flow downstream into rivers, lakes, and oceans, and they turn up when those water sources are treated or bottled for sale to consumers. If water isn't specifically treated to remove drugs, you may be taking them when you gulp from your allegedly healthy water bottle on that brisk hike in the hills.

They are also working their way down into the aquifers that are pumped to provide water to half the country. This is not a good thing.

Drugs do not necessarily need to be discarded on the expiration date on the drug company bottle or the prescription label. Pharmaceutical companies build a little extra time into expiration dates and the date on the pharmacy label is often simply a year from when it was dispensed. The official expiration date is when the company still guarantees the drug's full potency and safety, but it may still be effective much longer.

Fortunately, there are now a number of good options for safely disposing of drugs that are outdated or unneeded or both. This also includes OTC medications and vitamins or supplements. The best and easiest way to get rid of drugs is on National Prescription Drug Take Back Days, sponsored by the DEA and often operated through local police departments. Every April and October, you can gather up all those random bottles and tubes and turn them in, no questions asked. Call your local police department for info.

Some pharmacies provide drug disposal bins where you can also toss those bottles, and others offer prepaid systems to mail them to a drug disposal company. *DisposeMyMeds.org* can identify local places that will accept them.

If none of these options work for you, you can dispose of pills in the trash with a few precautions. Don't grind up pills or empty gel caps. Mix them with something people won't want to dig into, like used kitty litter or old coffee grounds. Then stick the nasty mess into a zipper bag or empty jar with a lid and toss it.

Every rule has exceptions.

The FDA recommends that certain very potent drugs, mostly painkillers, should be flushed no matter what. These are mostly drugs that could cause death or disaster if even the tiniest bit is ingested by a child or pet.

But don't flush anything else!

ASKING QUESTIONS

Wherever possible you should approach any proposed treatment or medication by looking at the Five Ws used in the world of journalism: Who? What? When? Where? Why? And don't move on with any treatment plan or medication until you are satisfied with the answers.

Who? Who is proposing or prescribing this? In a complex medical situation, there may be many players, and it's up to the patient and the caregiver to keep them straight and understand who's working on which parts of the problem. Who will actually perform or oversee the treatment? Where is this person and how soon can you see them?

What? Get as much specific information about the treatment plan or medication regimen as you can up front. Ask questions.

If you're having trouble communicating with the health care provider, back up and phrase the question differently. Be polite: *I'm having trouble understanding* is better than *You aren't making any sense.*

When? If the treatment plan involves a succession of steps, be sure you understand the timetable and order. How do these steps relate to each other? Must one be finished before the next can begin? How urgent is it to get started? Can anything be postponed?

Where? Most treatments will take place in locations other than the doctor's office. Find out where these are and plug them into your car's navigation system and your phone. (Or turn to the proper fold of the map.) Leave yourself extra time on your first visit. Make a dry run if you're dealing with a strange location and/or a crabby patient.

Why? This is probably the toughest question. You need to understand why a treatment is being proposed. What do they hope it will accomplish?

Not every illness will have a clearly defined line of treatment, and in some cases you may have more than one option. Ask more questions, but don't stall.

What is best? This is not always obvious. What is best for the patient may not be the suggested line of treatment. There are many reasons this could be true, including when a patient is failing and the prognosis is grim (*see* CHAPTER NINE: END OF LIFE ISSUES). Don't just assume that a suggested treatment is necessary. Doctors are trained and programmed to keep trying.

Sometimes the best treatment simply isn't available, whether through geography or cost or the fact that it is still experimental.

What is reasonable? Is this appropriate for the patient? What's the potential to do more harm than good? Is a treatment going to be really awful? What are you gaining if something will extend life for six months filled with dreadful side effects?

These can be very hard questions and there generally are not any right answers.

What is available? Most availability questions rise out of location. If you are in a geographically remote area, some options may require travel, including lengthy stays in an unfamiliar and more congested area.

If a treatment is new and only one person is performing it, there may be a significant time delay to get onto the medical conveyor belt. Does the time delay warrant the hope for a better outcome?

What is affordable? Far and away the worst possible situation is having insufficient financial resources in the middle of a major health crisis.

Ideally, the cost of a procedure or medication will be irrelevant because it's all covered. If you aren't in that situation, you still have choices, but they may not be good ones.

Is it worth doing something cheaper but less effective? Will time change the financial situation? Do you want to go into serious debt with the potential for bankruptcy?

All of these questions are terrible. May you never need to face them.

FIVE
THE PAPER JUNGLE

S ome people, it is rumored, enjoy paperwork. You probably don't see one of them when you look in the mirror. In fact, many folks purely hate any form of paperwork or bookkeeping or record keeping. Unfortunately, you usually don't have that luxury in a caregiving situation. It's vitally important to get on top of what needs to be done *right now* and have it completed yesterday.

Legal paperwork is one of those things that nobody likes to think about, much less do.

A will means that you're going to die. Advance directives mean that you're telling somebody to pull the plug. Why get involved with either? You intend to live forever in perfect health.

In addition to personal superstitions, family dynamics also come into play. Parents often don't want their children involved with (or aware of) their personal finances and don't provide information in an accessible way.

The flip side is just as common. Kids can't bear to think that Mom and Dad won't be around forever and are pretty sure that if they put their fingers in their ears and go *lalalalalala* they can avoid ever needing to consider the topic.

With all this avoidance floating around, it's no surprise that so few people have their legal paperwork in order.

We'll explain here what everybody should have and ways to put it in place for your personal situation. Keep in mind that the author is not an attorney and this should not be regarded as legal counsel.

Even if you are quite confident that everybody's affairs are in perfect order, flip through this section just in case you may have missed a little wrinkle. Little legal wrinkles can turn into big litigation creases when it's least convenient.

We are culturally conditioned not to talk about money or personal finance, but when somebody requires caregiving, there are almost always financial considerations. At the very least, routine bills need to be paid to keep the lights on. And at some point, a blizzard of explanations of benefits and bills from people you've never heard of will begin to hit your mailbox and inbox.

Sometimes financial issues are revealed as part of a quietly creeping problem, now suddenly at the heart of a crisis. Dementia, for instance. Or maybe things got into a muddle while your loved one was in denial about a physical problem. It can be challenging to figure things out.

But you need to do it and do it fast.

Major illness is itself very expensive. Costs are shocking even when they're expected and covered by insurance. For the uninsured or underinsured, they can be catastrophic.

Apart from the illness itself, the financial machinations are the least fun part of the entire experience.

LEGAL PAPERWORK

This is what people generally think of as "getting your affairs in order."

That sounds forbidding. It involves decisions you don't want to make about things you don't want to think about. Like dying, or lingering in a coma, or landing in the ER unconscious after being hit by an SUV.

It also sounds uncomfortable and expensive, probably involving lawyers. You can't avoid decision-making, but depending on the patient's situation and resources, you may not need an attorney at all.

You may get lucky and have a loved one with everything signed, sealed, and on record in the appropriate places. More likely, you'll need to scramble a little—either to find documents or to get them in place in a hurry.

Everything about legal paperwork is state-specific. You must have the appropriate information and forms and verbiage for the state where the patient lives.

If you also live in that state it's usually easier.

If you decide to use an attorney and the patient doesn't already have one, hire somebody who specializes in estate planning. Ask for referrals if possible. You're not saving money by using a lawyer who's cheaper, or fresh out of school, or a relative in a different state who'll be happy to help.

If you prefer not to use a lawyer, there are plenty of options, some better than others. Many free or inexpensive forms are online, but if you intend to handle your legal affairs on the internet, make sure you've got a reputable website and not just a slick one.

My recommendation is to start with *nolo.com* and use the relatively inexpensive WillMaker software available through Nolo and other booksellers. *Nolo.com* is an excellent clearing house for legal information and fill-in forms, and it's loaded with explanations and FAQs about whatever you're trying to do.

WillMaker features the necessary paperwork for every state, in the form and terminology those states require. It's easy and intuitive and asks lots of questions to be sure the correct information is all covered.

Making legal wishes official and valid also varies from state to state. Most documents require witnesses with no stake in the document. Some need to be notarized, which requires a licensed notary public. Some banks offer this service to customers at no charge, but if you need somebody to come to you, expect to pay an additional fee.

Advance Directives

These are crucial in a health care crisis.

Advance directives are written documents that state very clearly how the patient chooses to be treated, and who will make decisions if the patient isn't able to, for any reason. That person is usually known as the health care agent.

Different states have different names for these documents and for the people assigned to carry them out, another reason why it's important to have **state-specific forms** to ensure that they are valid. They are most commonly known as advance directives, living wills, or durable powers of attorney for health care. The term "durable" means it remains in effect when the person is incapacitated.

The health care agent has significant responsibilities, including hiring and firing medical personnel, signing hospital admission papers, authorizing treatments, and accessing private health care information.

HIPAA regulations are very specific about who can be told what, dating to the 1996 enactment of the Health Insurance Portability and Accountability Act. For the most part HIPAA provides excellent privacy protection, particularly in an electronic age. In health emergencies, however, it can complicate matters if you are not immediate kin to the patient. This has historically been an issue in domestic partnerships and same-sex marriages.

Some pre-printed advanced directive forms (sometimes available on the spot through health care facilities) offer a limited number of choices, usually couched in ambiguous terms such as "remain comfortable." Even these generally leave space to expand your wishes.

All advance directives include options for the type of care a patient wishes in different medical situations. Where a condition may be considered terminal, these start with two basic choices: prolong life for as long as possible or specify situations in which the patient does not wish to prolong life.

Here's where advance directives are crucial, because what the patient wants may not be what the patient's family has in mind. If Mom has signed a legal document stating that she does not want to be kept alive in specific instances and her children wish to keep her physical entity going in case a miracle cure shows up, Mom's wishes must prevail.

Advance directives usually go into effect when a doctor decides that a patient is incapacitated, but they can also be set up so that the health care agent has authority before that happens. In such cases, the patient's wishes always prevail.

Advance directives should be on file with all of the patient's doctors and provided on admission to any hospital or care facility. Even if you've taken this precaution, however, you may need to remind medical personnel that they *are* on file. If the patient uses dog tags or a medical alert device for other reasons, the info should also be on file with the managing company.

Advance care directives can be changed or rescinded at any time.

Do Not Resuscitate (DNR)

"Do not resuscitate" means exactly that: if the patient is not breathing or has no heartbeat, medical personnel should not attempt to revive them. It forbids cardiopulmonary resuscitation (CPR) but does *not* mean that the patient won't be treated for other medical issues, such as a broken bone.

DNRs tend to come into a medical situation when the patient is older and/or has been severely ill for quite some time with little likelihood of recovery.

They must be signed by a physician after discussion with the patient or by the health care agent.

Everybody takes a DNR seriously, but they need to know about it.

If the patient has a DNR, copies should be readily available to EMTs: on the refrigerator, bedside table, and/or any other obvious locations in the home. It should also be in the patient's purse or wallet (near medical insurance info) and in the caregiver's possession. It's also a good idea for everybody in the immediate caregiving circle to have PDFs on their phones.

Paramedics and ER personnel are trained to treat first and ask questions later. They are also trained to check for medical info immediately if there is a way to do so. EMTs look for medical alert jewelry and posted notifications in the home.

When a patient is transported to or from a nursing home or assisted living facility, the DNR should be on top of the accompanying paperwork, whether or not it applies to the current complaint.

A hospital will issue its own internal DNR when the patient is admitted. Be sure to ask about this. Once any kind of treatment is started it can be next to impossible to stop or reverse it.

A DNR can be revoked at any time. There is no form for this. You just need to tell the physician who signed it and destroy any existing copies.

Physician Orders for Life-Sustaining Treatment (Polst)

POLST is a relatively new and more specific medical document that clarifies the types of treatment a terminally ill patient wishes to have. It attempts to fill the space between the vagueness of many advance directives with the specificity of whether a patient wishes, for example, to forego antibiotics, intubation, or a feeding tube.

It does *not* mean that palliative care or treatment for non-life-threatening medical problems will be discontinued.

POLST requires a doctor's signature, supersedes DNR, and should be posted and carried in all the same places. It can also be revoked or changed at any time by consultation with the doctor.

Not all states have POLST. Check at *polst.org* to find out if it applies to you.

Conservatorship

If advance directives are not in place when a major medical event or accident occurs and the family does not agree on how matters should be handled, it may be necessary to have somebody designated as conservator for both medical and financial matters. This situation also arises for people who are disabled from birth.

In some cases, a person may specify their preferred conservator in advance, or may use an institution rather than a friend or relative.

Conservatorship is an unusual and complicated circumstance that may grow out of heated and irreconcilable disagreements. Court intervention and decisions mean attorneys, expenses, and a lot of time you could probably use better. Once the court is involved, it remains involved.

If you can possibly avoid this, you should.

Conflict Resolution

Formal or informal mediation may help to keep your family out of the court system while your loved one receives appropriate care in the absence of advance directives.

Remember that the goal is to handle matters *the way the patient would want to*. This is not always easy. If your family is in conflict, the disagreeing parties are likely to project their own wishes onto a patient who can't provide a thumbs-up or thumbs-down.

Start out with a family member as mediator at first if you've got somebody who gets along with everybody, is respected, and knows how to listen. Clergy are another excellent source for resolving family squabbles, provided that the parties in conflict hold similar religious views and the tenets of the religion are not in conflict with any of the proposed paths.

Professional mediation is sometimes available but can be costly. Also, unless everybody agrees in advance to abide by a mediator's advice, mediation may just eat up more time and money.

Durable Power of Attorney for Finances

Usually just called power of attorney, this legal document provides authority to make clearly specified financial decisions on behalf of somebody else. It may cover anything and everything or be limited to a single specific situation, such as the sale of a car. One person may designate multiple POAs for different situations.

POAs can be tailored to any possible situation or individual, but they should generally be given to people who have some business or financial expertise. The person given POA does not need to be a relative or close friend but should be good at getting things done.

Power of attorney can be revoked at any time when the person who granted it is of sound mind.

Nolo.com can tell you more than you will ever want to know about this complicated issue, which varies from state to state.

Wills and Trusts

The last will and testament figures in a lot of mystery fiction and television drama. It can be a dandy motive for nefarious behavior and lead to somebody being bumped off before the first commercial.

In real life, it's a lot more basic and fundamental and boring. Wills tend not to be written in disappearing ink, or burned except for one tiny scrap in a convenient fireplace, or challenged by a third cousin who's an artist in the Azores.

Everybody should have a will.

That's a lot easier to say than to enforce and by the time somebody dies, it is obviously too late.

Young adults think they'll live forever and older ones may recognize that it's a good idea, but since they're healthy right now, no rush and no worries. Every year, a lot of these people die and leave behind legal uncertainty and ambiguity, as well as some white-hot messes.

A very common excuse for not having a will is that it will all go to [fill in your blank here] anyway, so no big deal. Except that it *is* a big deal. Money and/or property are involved and the government has rules about the transfer of both.

Dying without a will is called **dying intestate** and it is a holy nightmare. If the person who passed away has significant resources, distant relatives and ex-spouses can start crawling out of the woodwork and complicate an already difficult situation. Even if the person had very little, there are still likely to be possessions and financial responsibilities of some sort.

You cannot leave government out of this by ignoring it.

The state *will* be involved, like it or not.

An estate's resources can be depleted significantly by the time matters get straightened out and assets are delivered to the beneficiaries.

In general, the intestate hierarchy of beneficiaries starts with the spouse, followed by children, parents, and siblings. Who gets how much and in what order may vary from state to state.

Living trusts are a more complex way to pass assets to beneficiaries and avoid probate, with tax implications and additional state-specific requirements. These are frequently used in larger or more complex estates but can also be helpful for the less wealthy. If you're confused by the distinctions, you're not alone. FAQs at *nolo.com* can help you determine whether this is a good option for your situation.

The bottom line is that something is better than nothing. That's true whether it's a scrap of paper right out of Agatha Christie or a deathbed video recorded on a cell phone.

THE WORLD OF HEALTH INSURANCE

Once upon a time, health insurance was fairly simple and straightforward. You got it through your job and it took care of most medical problems and hospitalizations. Matters were more complicated without insurance, but medical bills were fairly reasonable and it was often possible to negotiate payment when they weren't.

Those days are over.

Health insurance is far too large and complex a topic for this guidebook, so we'll simplify as much as possible.

In a complicated medical and/or insurance situation, you will probably still reach the distant shore, though it may take a while. Smooth sailing is not guaranteed.

The Affordable Care Act

To understand current health care specifics, we need to begin with the Affordable Care Act of 2010 (ACA), more commonly known as Obamacare. This was the first national legislation designed to make health coverage available to all Americans at a reasonable price, without discrimination by age, gender, or pre-existing conditions.

Under its original provisions, Americans were required to carry health insurance. If they had no coverage through work, they needed to take out a policy through a government exchange and report the information on their income tax. Consumers received discounts to make the policies actually affordable, and the federal government paid insurance companies to balance out any projected revenue losses created by being open to all.

Obamacare covered physical exams, mammograms, pregnancy, and prescription drugs. Children could be covered through the age of twenty-six on parental policies. Those at low income levels were covered through the expansion of Medicaid, with the federal government providing financial assistance to states for the increased costs.

The ACA went into full effect in 2014 against strong and bitter political opposition.

What's happened since then has been wide-ranging and inconsistent, starting with endless Congressional attempts to repeal the legislation. Beginning in 2017, new approaches to dismantling, deconstructing, and sometimes disemboweling the law's protections and procedures have come through executive orders or judicial challenges. All of this is subject to additional change with very little notice.

Bipartisanship in working out the United States version of universal health care has generally been in short supply. This is unlikely to change.

The writers of the original ACA compromised to achieve passage by omitting a public health option, which would have permitted any citizen to enroll in a government-controlled system like Medicare.

ACA Coverage

When Obamacare took effect, states were given the option to create their own insurance exchanges. These individualized exchanges allow residents to select policies with various levels of coverage offered by various private insurance companies.

Coverage for those in states without their own exchanges is handled on a national level, at *healthcare.gov*. Again, the companies and types of policies available vary by state and location. In some cases, they are quite limited.

This was a complex system from the beginning. Different policies were initially offered in different areas by different companies. The selection process ranged from daunting to nonexistent, since some areas offered only one choice. Insurance companies continued to call the shots.

Over time, insurers left various ACA markets, limiting choices and allowing those who remained to increase prices. At the same time, anything that raised health care costs for anything was likely to be blamed on Obamacare, whether a legitimate correlation could be made or not.

The ACA system limits open enrollment when anyone can

join to specific calendar periods. However, you can quality for a special enrollment period if you lose your existing health coverage, get married, have or adopt a child, or move.

Because the ACA is based upon the private health insurance industry, everything about its coverage has added layers to the medical world's bureaucratic underpinnings. This has significantly escalated endless paperwork, billing codes, and coverage confusion.

Private Health Insurance

Before the ACA, private insurance was the only option for those under sixty-five, and insurers could make whatever rules they wanted for individual policies.

Most rules related to pre-existing conditions, which were not looked on kindly. Pregnancy and prescription drugs were not automatically covered. Policies could be cancelled by the insurance company with little notice, pretty much whenever they felt like it.

Most private health insurance in the United States has always been provided through employers. The ACA did not change that system, though it added requirements that all policies must cover.

Employer-based insurance has long been popular because it is usually paid in part by the employer (who gets tax advantages), with the employee's payment portion automatically deducted from their paycheck. Having the employer choose the policy largely omits the complicated process of determining what type of coverage might be best for an individual, which is rarely a pleasant or easy process.

Sometimes an employer will offer a choice of policies. Usually this is between a PPO (preferred provider organization) or an HMO (health maintenance organization).

Private policies are also sometimes available that do not meet ACA requirements and are therefore cheaper. These don't cover everything and generally have very high deductibles. They are popular with the young, those who believe themselves medically invincible, and folks who can't afford anything else.

Private Retirement Policies

Some retirement benefit plans include health insurance. These policies are often similar to the pre-retirement health plan but may change over time. In general, when you have Medicare and one of these group retirement policies, Medicare pays first and the group pays second.

Confirm the terms and payment priorities of any such policy with your insurer.

COBRA Insurance

COBRA (Consolidated Budget Reconciliation Act) insurance policies allow you to keep the same coverage you have carried under a group health plan when you are no longer eligible for the benefits. Usually this occurs when you leave a job and don't yet have another. It is quite expensive, since the portion of the premiums that was paid by an employer is now also your responsibility. It is generally limited to eighteen months.

PPO or HMO?

Whether a preferred provider organization (PPO) or health maintenance organization (HMO) is better for you depends on where you live; your family's medical issues and history; your current care providers and how you feel about them; and whether you are willing to have your health care managed by a primary care physician (PCP).

If you have ongoing relationships with specific health care systems or providers who do not participate in an HMO program, then it makes sense to choose PPO coverage. With a PPO you generally pay a percentage of billed fees for service but can pick and choose your providers. Prescription coverage and deductibles included with a PPO plan will vary from one insurance company to another.

HMOs also may require deductibles, but they are usually flat rate and relatively low. A referral from your primary care physician is usually required to see a specialist, except in emergencies, and those referrals can take a while. You may have no choice of which specialist you see and will probably be expected to use the affiliated hospital.

Medicare

Medicare is government-issued health insurance for older Americans and some younger citizens with disabilities. As a "retirement" policy, it is available to the previously employed who have paid into the Medicare system through payroll deductions for at least ten years (forty quarters) over a lifetime of work. It may also be available to non-working spouses of covered individuals and, with additional payment, to those with no work history at all.

An individual of any age found eligible for Social Security Disability Insurance (SSDI) coverage, discussed below, will be entitled to Medicare coverage after the first two years of disability.

Medicare tends to be beloved by those who are enrolled. Health care agencies and providers don't like it as much, since the amounts paid for services are determined at the national level, though they may vary in different regions. All of them are a lot lower than what private insurance generally pays.

Medicare coverage has several possible components. One is automatic upon reaching the typical enrollment age of sixty-five and signing up. Others are optional. In some cases, not signing up upon first eligibility can lead to additional charges over the lifetime of coverage.

Medicare Part A is hospitalization insurance and is the cornerstone of every policy. It is mandatory, and those with the requisite work history get it for free.

Medicare Part B covers medical care other than hospitalization, including physicians, treatments, tests, procedures, and other medical charges. It is optional but will be added automatically to your Medicare Part A policy unless you opt out.

Part B carries a modest premium charge, which is deducted from your Social Security payment if you receive one. If you can possibly afford it, you should have this coverage.

Do not assume that other overlapping private or disability insurance will cover these costs if you get Medicare at any age. Check first with the carrier to avoid unpleasant surprises.

Medicare Part C is also known as **Medicare Advantage**. Medicare Advantage plans are offered by private companies and are designed to cover most medical expenses. They generally involve enrollment in an HMO of some sort and may require an additional fee. They usually have some copayments.

This coverage works by the government paying the insurance company a flat monthly fee to take over your Medicare contract. The insurer gambles that what they pay out on your behalf will be less than what the feds paid them for your contract. No matter how much care you receive, you will have no additional charges beyond those clearly spelled out in the contract.

Medicare Advantage plans may also include prescription drug coverage.

If you are happy with the HMO coverage attached to a Medicare Advantage plan, it is an excellent and economical option.

Medicare Part D is prescription drug coverage, available separately from many different companies. The best way to select a Medicare Part D policy is to work backward from the medications you are taking and see which ones are covered at the best rates for you.

Medicare is prohibited by law from negotiating with pharmaceutical companies, so you won't necessarily get your medications at the lowest possible rate.

Other Medicare options include **Medigap** or **Medicare Supplement** policies, which are written and billed separately by private companies. These policies are designed to cover the various copays and deductibles that may exist in your Medicare Parts A, B, and D policies. They are also complicated and require research.

The easiest way to determine your appropriate Medicare and additional coverage(s) is to consult an insurance agent *in your area* who is familiar with the available options and can tell you which ones work best with your current health care needs.

These agents get no fees from customers, and they can save you endless hours of confusing research and anguish, as well as quite a lot of money. And if your situation and needs change, they can help you find the new coverage you want.

Medicaid

Medicaid is a government program to provide health coverage for people with low income, high medical bills, and legal U.S. residency by citizenship or Green Card.

It is run by the individual states, which may or may not

choose to participate, and which can set their own eligibility standards beyond the basics. You will need to determine what your state requirements are for the specifics of your situation, particularly if there isn't any other health insurance. A social worker at the hospital can help set this up if the need for coverage results from an emergency.

ACA Medicaid coverage is available for those with income that falls below 133% of the federal poverty level. However, not all states opted to offer that coverage, and whether you can obtain coverage this way will depend on where you live.

Veterans Administration

Veterans of active military service are eligible for various types of health coverage through the Veterans Administration (VA). The types of benefits vary according to other eligibility factors such as income and service-related conditions. Most often someone depending upon VA coverage for the current caregiving situation already has some level of VA care.

Check *VA.gov* if you believe your uninsured or underinsured loved one is a veteran who might be eligible. Individual states also offer various types of veterans' health benefits.

PAYMENT ENCLOSED

Major illness is expensive, no matter who's paying. It's likely that several different players and business relationships are involved if you have private or government insurance.

You're considered self-insured and in deep manure if you don't have any coverage at all, as discussed below in the subsection on self-insurance.

But no matter who's involved, there will be financial issues and questions, even if you have buckets of money and no major problems with health care or health care providers.

Coverage Disputes

One consistent area of contention are charges that pop up because somebody who did something is **not in your network**. This is most common in situations starting in the emergency room. If emergency surgery is involved, it's almost a foregone conclusion. In matters of life and death, nobody has the time or inclination to research whether the anesthesiologist is on your insurance plan's list.

Balance billing is a related issue that varies from place to place. It occurs when a doctor or other provider bills the patient for the part of the original bill not covered by insurance. It is illegal for Medicare providers and regulated or forbidden in some states.

Occasionally you will have to do battle.

You can sometimes win these battles by persistence and civility. Other times you will want to bang your head against the wall. Occasionally you will make it through a telephone tree to a real person who has access to the file. If you need to come back later, you will—eventually—be connected with a *different* real person who will ask you the same questions again. And so on.

Be calm. Persevere. Medical bills are almost always negotiable at some level. That level may not be yours, but it's worth a try.

Another area loaded with minefields is prescription drug coverage.

Most insurance carriers have a **formulary** that lists the medications that your policy covers and the consumer's payment requirement for each. These are complicated lists that vary from one insurance company to another, one region to another, and one year to another.

Doctors prescribe medications they believe are appropriate. If the insurance carrier disagrees and doesn't cover something, ask the doctor if something cheaper will achieve the same desired results.

This problem frequently arises with very new and/or very expensive drugs, the ones advertised on TV. Sometimes the doctor will prescribe these new meds after being badgered to do so by the patient.

Ask your doctor if medical advice from a television commercial is right for you.

Experimental treatments and procedures (or those your insurance company considers experimental) may not be covered. In some instances, this may involve ongoing clinical trials; in others, the treatment might be regarded as flat-out quackery.

In either case, if you've tried everything else and you're prepared to wage war, get ready to be stonewalled, at the cost of much personal time and angst.

How Medical Prices Are Determined

The short answer is: "Who knows?" There is, however, a system of sorts.

The "rack rate," or alleged charge for medical services, is aimed at the highest-possible-paying customer. A potentate with his own island empire and a rare blood disorder, for example, or a rock star who banged his throat in a bungee-jumping accident.

Some medical consumers pay this rate, no questions asked. They are precious few.

The charges for all medical services and procedures start with some version of the same inflated billing scheme. As it moves in your direction, it begins to resemble a giant financial spider web, with your loved one the tender morsel trapped in its intricate and sticky trap.

Hospitals begin their billing with what is known as a **chargemaster**, and every hospital (or hospital group) has its own version.

The chargemaster lists up to 50,000 services and procedures and items that a patient may be charged for during a hospital stay. The rack rate or negotiating starting point for each of these items is calculated and listed.

The existence of chargemasters only became publicly known in 2013. They are supposed to be available to consumers. You may or may not be able to easily see a copy of a hospital's chargemaster, but you'll learn what's in it when you start getting bills.

Two hospitals may sit side-by-side and offer the same general range of services. However, their different chargemasters probably list very different costs for the same things. A physician affiliated with more than one hospital probably won't know the difference.

Outside of a hospital, other health care providers also have set rates that they charge for various procedures. These differ from practice to practice and facility to facility.

What Does It *Really* Cost?

In general, nobody expects to get paid those inflated amounts.

This leads us to step two in the price determination derby, wherein doctors, medical groups, hospitals, and most other health care providers cut their own deals with insurance companies and each other.

Doctors, hospitals, and other providers want to be paid as much as they can. Insurance companies want to pay the smallest amount they can. It's the middle ground between these extremes that gets complicated.

Insurance carriers make side deals with care providers and institutions, establishing the rates that their customers will actually be charged. Larger companies, or those with a large population in a particular area, can usually make better deals than smaller ones. But they all start with the inflated numbers designated as the "cost" of the procedure or service. Here is where you run into the $28 Tylenol and the $43 disposable diaper.

Depending on the terms of these side deals and the policies of the billing institution and your own insurance coverage, you may be responsible for paying the difference between what was billed and what was paid on your behalf.

Other complications can arise, particularly for those who have gambled on high-deductible plans for lower premiums. Those deductibles must be met before other major benefits can kick in, and those benefits may or may not actually cover the expenses incurred.

A lot of this billing and paying and paperwork and negotiation will occur in the background from the very beginning, but you won't necessarily be aware of any of it for at least a couple of months.

Nor are you likely to care. You're preoccupied with making sure that your loved one gets the best care and treatment that's humanly possible. You also are juggling a mountain of other surprise responsibilities, like notifying people and explaining to work why you need more time off.

Self-Insurance

If you have no insurance at all, you are euphemistically referred to as "self-insured." This means that you are responsible for every single penny yourself, at the rack rate. This status sets off alarms in an ER's billing system that quickly translate into actions.

Nobody can be turned away from the emergency room. That's the law.

But you may shortly be moved to a county or other government hospital whether you want to go or not. There, hospital personnel and social workers will probably assist you to obtain potential coverage through the VA or Medicaid if you meet the requirements. They may also be able to steer you toward other financial assistance.

Explanations of Benefits

Explanations of benefits (EOBs) are required by law to inform you of:

- What you have been charged
- What adjustments may have been made to those charges
- What exclusions may apply
- What sections and codes are involved
- Your financial responsibility for these expenses

EOBs are not bills, but rather a head-on collision between bureaucratic legalese and the free enterprise system.

EOBs also arrive long after the services have been provided, but frequently before other involved players make their payments to one another. When you get one related to a hospital stay, sit down before opening it.

A great deal of coding goes into medical billing and payment, and one tiny error somewhere along the way can set off an avalanche of subsequent problems. This is one reason why it's a good idea to keep track of these as they come in and to keep them all together. But don't let them paralyze you. Remember, they are *not* bills. The bills will come separately and be an entirely different kind of interpretive headache.

As we all know, if any part of the health care system thinks you owe them money, they will definitely be in touch.

Other Benefits

It's hardly an advantage, but serious injury or illness can actually kick off a useful series of financial events that will help. Often this involves policies or funds that you've paid into for a long time without really thinking about it. These are likely to vary from state to state and location to location, but they're worth checking out anywhere.

Disability payments provide funds to offset the lost income that a major medical event may cause. They often come through the state or through a municipality or government agency for which you work.

Short-term disability coverage takes effect after a specified period of time and will usually be initiated by your employer once it's clear that you're going to be disabled for a while. Short-term disability is renewed at brief intervals to avoid abuse.

Sometimes this coverage will gradually morph into **long-term disability coverage** with longer renewal periods. This is not the same as long-term care insurance, which is used to offset payments for caregiving (*see* CHAPTER EIGHT: MOVING ON).

Some people carry private disability policies specific to their own work or professional situation. Other policies through work or affiliation groups may also provide benefits, particularly if an accident was involved.

Social Security Disability Insurance

Receiving longer-term disability payments may require applying for Social Security Disability Insurance (SSDI). This federal program provides payment to those who have paid into the Social Security system through payroll taxes.

To be eligible, you must have a disability that will continue for at least a year or that is likely to result in death within a year. Like many government processes, this one is complex and can take a long time to implement. SSDI coverage is coveted and subject to considerable abuse. Many first-time applicants are denied, which requires appeals and sometimes hiring a specialist attorney.

When approved, retroactive benefits will be paid to the date of first eligibility.

SSDI recipients are also eligible to receive Medicare coverage, beginning two years after the date of first eligibility.

Accidents

If the current medical situation is the result of an accident, you'll find additional hurdles and paperwork to negotiate.

If the accident occurred in a public or private facility (including private homes), liability insurance will almost certainly become involved. If some form of public transportation is related, the associated municipalities (often self-insured) will be responsible for liability.

Accidents resulting from automobiles or other vehicles with wheels and/or motors move into other specific categories. An auto accident between two vehicles will often bring together two different insurance companies representing the drivers—along with police reports, eyewitness accounts, weather conditions, and a host of other issues.

If your loved one can be considered responsible for the accident and there are other injuries, these insurance claims immediately leap to a more complicated level.

Sometimes accident claims can be resolved quickly and easily by adjustors who work for the insurance companies involved and know the current "market value" of such claims in your area.

If that doesn't happen, expect lawyers to become players and lawsuits to be filed.

When you are approached by attorneys wishing to represent your loved one, be very careful before making representation agreements. You have time to do this right, and you should start by discussing it with your own insurance carrier and anybody on your caregiving team with legal experience.

This type of litigation tends to drag out and will always be simmering on a back burner of the medical crisis.

A serious accident that was somebody else's fault tends to start dollar signs floating through the air. Friends and relatives may entertain visions of large sums of money dropping out of insurance heaven right into your loved one's lap.

Try to be careful and thoughtful about all of this. There's a fine line between getting what you are entitled to and raw greed.

NON-MEDICAL EXPENSES

A major medical event does not create a moratorium on routine living expenses. You may be dealing with all sorts of medical issues and related problems, but in the meantime, the rent and electricity and car insurance and everything else that is associated with day-to-day life continues.

If you are caring for somebody who has been living alone and handling these matters, the situation is doubly challenging, even if everything has been handled capably and correctly. If the patient has limited means, it's important to get on top of it quickly.

If your loved one is able to cooperate, everything will be much easier, though you still may meet with resistance. Acknowledging that one can't handle their own affairs is a sad and daunting realization. Sharing personal finances feels like—and is—an invasion of privacy.

It's usually a good idea to stress that this is just a temporary arrangement until your loved one is able to take care of business again. And to be gentle but firm when you broach the subject.

If the patient is not conscious or capable of making decisions or arrangements, everything becomes exponentially more complicated. You may need to have somebody appointed by a court as conservator (discussed above) in order to keep the lights on.

Start by deciding who is the best person on your caregiving team to take on financial matters and have that person added as a signatory to any bank accounts involved in billpaying. This person doesn't even need to be geographically accessible once you set things up. And they may not have any other caregiving responsibilities beyond communicating with the primary caregiver.

The best possible solution is to have your loved one sign a durable power of attorney (POA) to handle specifically designated financial affairs. At the same time, the POA designee needs free rein to go through personal files to determine the patient's financial obligations.

Everything will be much simpler if you can continue working with the patient's existing bank accounts. These are already established and may also be set up for direct deposits and direct payment withdrawals. If the patient hasn't already done so, establish online payments when possible. A lot of this can be done directly through the bank account, and a bank officer can walk you through the procedure if you need help.

Be aware of payments that may come due at longer intervals, such as insurance premiums, IRS quarterly payments, license renewals, and property taxes.

If the patient is likely to take over these responsibilities again, try not to make too many changes to the established systems, even if they are contrary to how you would do things for yourself.

If things are seriously out of control, with significant debts and other financial problems, it's smart to consult a nonprofit credit counselor. These people are trained to help work out a consolidation plan for outstanding bills and a system going forward for bills to come. Finding one locally is usually a better solution than pulling an 800 number off a late-night TV ad.

If it's *really* a mess, consider consulting a bankruptcy attorney, POA in hand. There is usually no charge for an initial consultation, and you will emerge with a much clearer sense of how much financial trouble your loved one is in. It may turn out that bankruptcy is not the necessary solution, but you will almost certainly gain useful information and might also get input on how to fix matters short of actual bankruptcy.

If the IRS is pounding on the door and there isn't any obvious way to satisfy them quickly, consult a CPA or an enrolled agent (EA). Enrolled agents are authorized by the US Department of the Treasury to handle IRS matters, either through IRS examinations or previous experience as an IRS employee. EAs know all the ins and outs and shortcuts to getting your loved one's obligation stripped down to what is actually owed, not what the IRS may be claiming is owed.

Spoiler alert: these two figures are rarely the same.

SIX
THE DAILINESS OF DAILY LIFE

I n any long-term or chronic caregiving, life generally slides
into an equally long-term and chronic set of patterns and activities. Here is where everybody begins to face challenges there
wasn't time to adequately process previously.

One challenge may be that things are not getting much better and may not be likely to. You thought you were waiting for
stability, but this is not the stability you had in mind. The same
is likely true for the patient, only more so.

Hope is a great motivator and energizer, but it wears thin
after a while. When the medical future is uncertain, you can look
ahead to better times, or at least less difficult ones. You can pray
and cross your fingers and hold good thoughts.

But when the patient plateaus at a level that nobody is ex-
cited about, it becomes a lot tougher to spread that smile across
your face and greet each coming day.

So where does everybody go from here?

DAY AFTER DAY AFTER DAY
Step back and assess your overall situation.

In the beginning there probably wasn't time for such con-
templation, because you were busy juggling chainsaws and call-

ing people and trying to figure out what you were going to do next. The next hour, that is—not the next week or month or year.

Often things get set up in a certain way during that initial period and then stay locked in place through inertia and habit.

That's one thing you're looking for.

Can something in the daily routine(s) be done more efficiently or effectively? What's no longer necessary but continues through habit? What might make anybody or everybody more comfortable?

Look at your daily schedule as well as your loved one's. Did you make major changes in your circadian rhythms or dietary habits or viewing preferences? Did the patient? Are these changes useful and valid, or a pain in the butt?

If they're useful, look at why and aim at more of the same. If not, think about how to establish or revert to better habits.

For instance, if everybody is eating more soup and fewer cookies, you're on a good pathway. If the customary deep-fried everything isn't an easy option, your arteries can only be happier for the break. If you're using less caffeine and staying awake, keep it up. If anybody or everybody is drinking less alcohol, congratulate yourselves.

There's a flip side, of course. Are there more bags of chips in the cupboard? Six kinds of ice cream? Do you always hit the burger joint on your way home? Is it easier to get to sleep with a slug of booze at bedtime? Be honest with yourself.

Look also at the patient's physical setup.

Would it help to move the bed or bring in a different chair? Is there a better tray table configuration than what you're using? How about a sickroom minifridge? Or renting a hospital bed?

What about moving the patient down to the living room? If this is going to continue for a long time, everybody might be happier that way and it would be easier to accommodate visitors.

If the patient is getting up and moving independently, have you removed the throw rugs and rickety little tables? Are there plenty of automatic nightlights set up for evening bathroom visits? Nighttime pathways should blaze like an airport runway.

See CHAPTER EIGHT: THE NEW NORMAL for specific ways to adapt the living space.

And keep thinking, on a day-to-day basis, about how you can improve anything and everything.

Let the Patient Win Sometimes

It's easy to forget how helpless your loved one feels. The dailiness will get to them, too. Make a point of letting them win from time to time when there's a non-medical decision to make. If you're bossy by nature, caregiving brings that front and center.

Pay attention. Listen.

And consider how you'd feel in a world where you've lost all control.

Medical Alert Systems

Medical alert jewelry is an excellent idea for anybody with a chronic condition who leaves home for any reason or who is sometimes alone and may need to summon help. This doesn't need to be clunky and obvious. Many reasonably stylish variants are available, and a bracelet, necklace, or dog tag is best.

Someone with serious ongoing health issues doesn't want anybody providing incorrect emergency care if they get hit by a bus or lose consciousness in public.

Paramedics automatically look for this jewelry. It doesn't need to have intimate medical details printed on it, but can simply provide an 800 number to call, or note a basic diagnosis or life-threatening allergy.

In general, you're better off with a system that charges a small monthly fee for telephone access.

ACTIVITIES FOR ONE AND ALL

Few activities are as stultifying as lying in a sickbed for days or weeks on end.

Figuring out how to pass the time is important for any kind of prolonged caregiving. Get on top of it before it gets on top of the patient and everybody else.

If you know the patient really well, you already have a pretty clear idea of what will and won't work to fill those long hours of healing and recovering. Otherwise, this may take a bit of detective work.

Activities for the patient depend on three interrelated elements: the physical ailment, the patient's temperament, and what the patient normally enjoys.

Reading

Reading is a favorite pastime for patients of all ages. This can be a good time for both patient and caregiver to catch up on the latest from a favorite author, tackle Russian literature, or whittle down a stack of aging magazines.

If holding a book is a problem, try a lightweight e-reader or other electronic device, which can also enlarge the print to a more comfortable reading size. E-books may also be read on a smart phone, tablet, laptop, or desktop computer.

E-books are simple to download, and once you buy them, they're yours for good. Material in the public domain (no longer under copyright) may be available for free. Check with the local library to learn their procedures for borrowing e-books.

Trouble concentrating on the printed page? Try audio books and listen to the same material in either abridged or unabridged form. These are also available through most public libraries. Earbuds are important unless you're listening together intentionally.

Comfort reads are invaluable in times of illness and stress.

Reading is a pastime *for the reader*. There is no requirement that it improve, inform, or uplift. Re-reading J.K. Rowling or Agatha Christie may transport your loved one back into safe and familiar worlds. There's a reason that popular fiction is popular. People like it.

Comfort reads also tend to be lengthy, so a reader can get lost in them for a while. Many come from prolific authors, sometimes as part of a lengthy series.

A patient who normally reads nonfiction is likely to have very definite preferences. Pay attention and provide things they specifically want or request. Don't try to guess, because you'll probably be wrong.

Magazines are rapidly disappearing from the national landscape, and subscriptions are often absurdly cheap. Newspapers are also evaporating, but available in print at *higher* rates than before. Nearly all printed news media are also available online at relatively low cost.

Television and Visual Media

Some people like the comfort and background noise of a television running much of the time. Some are addicted to cable news. Some prefer all sports, all the time. Some will happily watch whatever may be running when they turn on the set. Some set equipment to watch favorite shows at a more convenient time. Some watch specific programs and need to view them uninterrupted from the beginning. Some binge-watch.

No matter how you and your loved one are accustomed to watching TV, you probably both have fairly consistent habits. If those happen to intersect, consider yourself lucky. If they don't, the patient's wishes have priority in the sickroom. Noise-cancelling headphones can be a mental lifesaver.

You may want to add a small TV and a new cable connection in the sickroom if that's the activity center for a while. Position a remote near the patient's dominant hand and you're done.

In addition to the hundreds of stations available through many cable companies, you can probably watch all manner of current movies, limited series, and network series on demand through your regular setup, sometimes for a small additional fee, or through a streaming service.

Streaming has the added advantage of starting whenever you want, taking a break when you choose, and then coming back later exactly where you left off.

Just about everything that has ever been produced for film or television is now available on DVD. DVDs are going out of fashion, but billions are still loose in the world. And if the patient's viewing equipment no longer includes a DVD player, they are also incredibly cheap.

I Love Lucy. The Godfather. Seinfeld. The Original Mickey Mouse Club. The Sopranos. Game of Thrones. M*A*S*H.

You get the drift.

Games

People either love or hate games.

If the patient enjoys them, you have the potential for endless hours of entertainment. Somebody who likes online games will already have continuing favorites, so your role is simple and straightforward. Make sure the equipment used to play them is available. Then quietly back out of the room.

If the patient does a lot of video gaming online, make sure that their preferences are in line with their new medical realities.

Games that involve bright flashing lights, for example, can trigger a seizure in somebody with new brain issues. If you aren't sure about this, check with the medical team. You don't want to learn this the hard way.

Somebody who prefers old fashioned board games is likely to have a stack of favorites. If they are already in a group that plays games regularly, consider inviting the others to do a version of this in the sickroom.

And if there's a game with an element of nostalgia that you think could be fun, you can probably go online and find exactly the same edition of Monopoly from when you were kids.

Puzzles

If the patient normally enjoys puzzles, all kinds of wonderful options require little exertion. For those who find puzzles of all sorts frustrating, don't even try.

If the patient enjoys jigsaw puzzles, you're really in luck.

There may already be a stash in a closet, or you can ask people to get them when they wonder how they can help. They're cheap in thrift shops. Even purchased new, it's worth every penny to keep your loved one content and occupied. Jigsaws are also available to work online, frequently for free.

Jigsaws also help with visitors. Visitors often have no idea what to do or say, especially during the first shocked visit or two. A jigsaw on a card table can function as a diversion and icebreaker, making it more likely they'll return.

Printed puzzles are portable and can be set aside and resumed later. This includes crosswords, sudoku, word search, anagrams, matching, cryptograms, acrostics, logic, and math puzzles. All are also available online.

In some cases of brain damage, patients may be instructed to work certain types of puzzles as part of their occupational therapy. If the patient has difficulty, or doesn't like puzzles to start with, or is just feeling ornery, the caregiver may need to force the issue. Nicely.

Not advised: *The doctor said you need to do those word searches, so get to it or you'll never get better.* Better: *C'mon, let's get going on today's word searches. Twenty minutes, and then we'll take an Oreo break.*

Music

Almost everybody likes music, which has the delicious capacity to change and improve their mood almost instantly.

Some people like only a narrow range of music, while others have broad and comprehensive tastes. If the patient's preferences are similar to your own, consider yourself very lucky and set up a good sound system in the sickroom. This can be as simple as a smartphone with a wireless speaker.

Cumbersome music systems with a lot of physical equipment and speakers are less popular these days, but if that's what your loved one has, figure out how to use it and don't complain. If you're out of your element here, find somebody in your broader caregiving circle who can help.

Simply turning on the radio can provide a perfectly gratifying musical background. The radio also allows a switch from jazz to bluegrass simply by changing stations.

If you're an opera fan and the patient loves country, get noise-cancelling headphones.

BREAKING OUT: GREAT ESCAPES

A patient who's improving is likely to get restless and a little stir crazy.

So is the caregiver. We all sometimes yearn to escape.

It can be a huge psychological boost for the patient to get out of the house briefly. Maybe this will be as simple as sitting out in the yard on a sunny day or walking to the mailbox. Have them take baby steps and do it with a spotter. Try not to hover but stay close enough to break a fall and by all means offer an arm.

As a patient improves, medical instructions usually include beginning to exercise. If the patient's previous notion of exercise was bench-pressing the recliner lever, a slow start is essential.

Even if the patient was previously running marathons, it can take some serious readjustment to get used to the new way their body wants to work. *Everybody* needs to take it easy at first, even Olympians. Physical achievers are most likely to push themselves too hard too quickly.

If the patient now uses assistive devices—a wheelchair, walker, crutches, a cane—a whole world of psychological issues looms on the horizon.

Only old people need this... A walker? That's ridiculous... I'm fine, just fine, really!... I look like my mother/father/Great Aunt Edna... This can't be me... Will I ever walk/run/swim/golf/ play tennis again?

Begin with simple things that the patient can manage right now. Maybe start with chair exercises. Get one of hundreds of available easy exercise or yoga or Pilates videos or find on-line classes. If the weather's okay, your loved one can build up strength systematically by walking one house farther each time they go out. Access to a swimming pool offers a great way to manage non-weight-bearing exercise.

After a while, the patient may move into a more advanced or complicated exercise program. Or not.

No matter how slow the progress, something is always better than nothing.

Field Trips

Going out into the world can also involve destinations that are just plain fun. If they're excursions you also enjoy, even better. If not, maybe you can recruit someone else from the extended caregiving team with a mutual interest.

Be realistic about what your loved one can handle and plan everything out in advance. Build in lots of extra time and don't be too ambitious. Start with something you know they want to do. If somebody is recovered enough to realize that they desperately need a haircut, that's a fine start. Or a mani-pedi. Or a massage.

Grooming can build self-confidence, which is often shaky after a medical event. When you look better, you feel better.

The patient might not be ready for a major league baseball game, but you could watch Little League at the local park. Live theater may be beyond reach but go see a matinee at a local movie theater. Not ready for the art museum? How about a gallery?

If the patient is on a recovery plateau, watch the sunset at the beach rather than walking along the shore. Go to lunch someplace casual, with a menu that won't throw anybody's digestive system out of whack.

Be prepared to cut anything short with little or no notice.

Travel

How will travel fit into the patient's new life? Mostly that depends on how travel fit into the patient's previous life.

A homebody isn't likely to suddenly yearn to visit Tasmania, and an inveterate traveler won't want two weeks in even the nicest timeshare. The trick is to find something relatively easy, affordable, and compatible with your loved one's notion of holiday.

A destination is better than a road trip. If seeing friends or relatives is part of that destination, make sure they're okay with the plan. You're likely to need more host attention than usual.

Where young grandchildren are involved, a nearby hotel room is a smart investment. In fact, hotels are a good idea when visiting anybody besides true intimates.

It's always nice to have somewhere to retreat where you can lock the door and put out a "Do Not Disturb" sign. Get a quiet, ground-floor room and ask about handicap accommodations when you make reservations. Call the hotel directly rather than going through a website.

If you haven't already done this, have the doctor approve a disabled license plate or placard. These can usually be used in other states, but check requirements in advance.

Figure on accomplishing about half of what you set out to do. Be proud if you hit that mark. Be ready to stop something early or take a day off and hang out at the hotel. Try not to overbook activities or over plan anything.

Leaving the country isn't a great idea for somebody with a serious medical problem. Without family reasons to go abroad, everything will be easier if you stay in the United States.

If your loved one is determined to travel abroad, plan as much as possible in advance and don't expect to do a lot of running around or eating in fancy restaurants. Consider a river cruise so you can be based in the same room through the entire trip, with optional side trips.

Do plenty of research about who pays for what if you run into health issues while abroad.

Bring extra medications and copies of all prescriptions. Be realistic about how much equipment you'll need. Most adults in need of care require as much paraphernalia as newborn babies.

For a patient traveling alone, get doctor's notes so you can accompany them to the gate and have the folks on the other end meet them at the jetway. Order airport wheelchairs in advance and arrange for special meals and preboarding as necessary. Let the gate agent know your loved one may require special help.

Be sure that everybody involved at every stage of the journey knows both the overview and their specific parts in the process. You do not want any weak links in this chain.

Finally, get travel insurance! It's not cheap, but the peace of mind is priceless.

Holidays

Holidays are benchmarks for most of us, no matter which ones we celebrate.

Serious illness shakes all that up, making a mockery of the idea of gathering with loved ones in a time of shared joy.

If you're coming up on an important holiday, lay the groundwork well in advance to quietly streamline and restructure activities. Make a point of saying it's just for this one year, even if you have to cross your fingers.

Don't pretend everything will be the same, because it won't be. And underlying everything may be a shared (though usually unspoken) realization that this could be the last time.

If the patient has traditionally been at the heart of holiday celebrations, having that change abruptly can be difficult and heart wrenching for all. Sometimes the hardest hit is a perfectionist patient who knows that they'd be able to do a much better job of everything.

Simplify. Cut the guest list. We learned in the pandemic that sometimes holiday plans can and should be changed, even when nobody wants to.

Major holidays usually involve food. Keep in mind that it's possible to order a complete meal from many grocery stores, leaving only one or two "mandatory" family dishes to be prepared.

Changing locations can be an easy and effective solution.

Go to another relative's place for Passover Seder. Make reservations for Thanksgiving dinner at the zoo or a local restaurant.

You may get some open-ended invitations—*We'd love to have you join us*—but think them through before you agree. It might seem nice to visit relatives, or an old friend, but only if it won't be more trouble than it's worth.

If decorating is usually part of the holiday in question, cut things back.

Christmas is especially difficult because many folks add decorations over the years without actually getting rid of anything they already have. If an entire corner of the basement is stuffed with Christmas decorations, figure out which ones are most meaningful and don't bring the rest of it out.

Skip the outdoor lights unless the Scouts are going to put them up and take them down. You don't need every single ornament on the tree, and maybe you don't even need the tree. Get a little one and put it on a table with a handful of special ornaments. Or skip the tree altogether and get a poinsettia the size of a washing machine.

Music is the easiest part of a holiday to maintain. Keep it playing.

Figure out ways the patient can participate. If they love giving the neighborhood kids candy at Halloween, maybe they can sit near the door and watch as somebody else fills the trick-or-treat sacks.

Focus on what's still happy about the holiday or holiday season, even if you routinely retreat to the bathroom for a good cry. Holidays can be physically exhausting as well as emotionally enervating. You need to treat yourself well.

If you're the one orchestrating holiday changes, build in a couple of things that will give you pleasure. You deserve it.

FAITH ISSUES

What exactly constitutes a religious or faith community? It can be anything from a massive cathedral to a gathering by the river. Here it refers to any group of people who share a spiritual belief system.

According to the Pew Research Center, 70.6% of the American public identify as Christian, including 25.4% Evangelical Protestant, 14.7% Mainline Protestant, and 20.8% Catholic. Non-Christian Faiths make up only 5.9% and include Jewish, Muslim, Buddhist, Hindu, and our old friend, Other.

Where the statistics get interesting is the Unaffiliated category, which comprises 22.8% and includes not just Atheists

(3.1%) and Agnostics (4.0%) but also our other old friend in religion discussions: None.

Historically, wars have been fought over religion, quite a lot of them.

You want to avoid starting any more during your own caregiving experience.

This isn't always easy.

Some families have awkward differences of opinion about whose God expects what. If some people in the equation don't believe in *any* deity, that can be a major problem for others who are certain those people are on the road to eternal damnation.

Major illness also brings a lot of buried religious beliefs, feelings, and resentments out of hibernation. Belief systems run deep, even when someone has come to challenge or disregard them.

And there's no way around it: serious injury or illness forces people to think about death. Which they *really* don't want to do.

You can't assume that all members of the patient's family have the same beliefs or attitudes. Even if this is your very own family. Unity of belief may be more likely in some faith communities, but there are always rebels.

Now may seem like the perfect opportunity to share your own faith, but people understand their own beliefs and generally hold them strongly. Don't push for conversion to another faith, or for belief to a nonbeliever, no matter how badly you want to. Holding back can be very difficult and stressful, particularly if recovery is not imminent.

If containing your anxiety about the patient's nonbelief is too difficult, share it with your own religious leaders.

It is also a terrible idea to have religious disagreements or discuss the nature of afterlife in the presence of the patient unless the patient initiates the conversation. This is true whether or not the patient appears to be conscious. There are far too many reports from people who overheard their condition and prognosis discussed in grim and gory detail while they appeared to be unaware of their surroundings. Watch what you say!

The patient's religious beliefs must take priority. Period.

Do not bring any religious visitors to the patient unless they agree in advance. A person who's too sick to get out of bed isn't in any shape to ask somebody to leave them alone or to show unwanted guests to the door.

A member of the family or caregiving team who's convinced that the eternal soul of the patient is at risk may present that case concisely *once.* After that, leave it alone unless the patient brings it up.

Most hospitals have chaplains available for different faiths, and these clergy are likely to show up at some point in the patient's room. Once back home, however, meeting spiritual needs can be more complicated.

Someone who regularly attends religious services may acutely feel the lack of that connection during prolonged periods of illness and recovery. Meeting that need may be as simple as tuning in to religious programming on TV or radio or listening to gospel music.

Some religious communities have continued the remote options established during COVID-19 shelter-in-place orders because they are relatively easy to maintain and—more importantly—allow people to participate who might otherwise be shut out.

If your loved one's faith community doesn't offer that option and the patient isn't healthy enough to attend in person, request that ordained and lay members of the church leadership visit regularly.

When the patient starts feeling better and wishes to attend in person, be sure that there are available accommodations. This might mean space for a wheelchair, or a seat on the aisle in the back, or even looking on from the crying room if the patient isn't yet comfortable being out in the community. One longtime member of my own church attended services on a gurney after a stroke limited his mobility.

Arrive early so you have plenty of time to settle in and *ask for help* any time it's needed. You will never be in a space more geared toward assisting the faithful.

Plan your escape as well. You may not wish to stay for coffee hour, for instance. If you want to slip out just before services end, ask an usher for help in advance. And if the patient grows weary or runs out of steam midway through the service, make as graceful an exit as possible without apology.

Respect for the patient's beliefs and privacy doesn't mean you can't be praying your own heart out, however.

Thank and encourage anybody who wants to pray on behalf of your loved one, whether or not you share their beliefs. "Thoughts and prayers" is a term that gets abused, but it's important. Even when you're certain you're on the one true path, others feel just as fervently that their own paths are correct.

Always be gracious to anyone who offers prayers, thoughts, or good wishes of any sort. Sending positive energy into the universe can only help.

SEVEN
CARING FOR THE CAREGIVER

Who's taking care of *you?*

Caregivers often get short shrift because what they do doesn't look difficult or complicated to outsiders. We know better.

Always keep in mind the instruction you're given on airplanes: *Put your own mask on first before helping others.* Don't think of self-care as a chore or an act of selfishness. Ever.

If you aren't at the top of your form—or are barely struggling to stay in the middle of your form—you'll be less effective as a caregiver and more miserable as a person. Keeping yourself healthy, rested, and calm creates a better atmosphere for everyone.

Start small.

Take a break, brew a pot of tea, and drink the first cup by yourself in the kitchen. If you're worried that you'll miss something in the sickroom, set up a baby monitor so you'll hear any problems.

Spritz on a little cologne, so long as you know it won't bother or nauseate the patient.

Find a comfortable chair in another part of the home or shut yourself in the bathroom for five minutes with a favorite magazine. After a day or two, if the world hasn't ended, make it ten minutes. Work up to fifteen and then start doing it twice a day.

Walk around the block. If that feels like too much, walk to the mailbox and back, then a few houses down the block, then to the corner. Keep the timeframe short enough so you don't keel over from anxiety but long enough to appreciate taking a deep breath on a beautiful day. Or splashing through puddles if it's raining.

A napping patient won't even miss you.

If they're awake, put your cell phone in your pocket and their phone at their side and set it to speed dial your number. If they can't or won't use a cell, look into old-style walkie talkies and wear something with bigger pockets.

Buy yourself a box or bag of your favorite candy and don't share it with anyone. If the patient enjoys ice cream, get a container of the flavor you like as well as the one they do. Maybe with a jar of hot fudge sauce and a can of whipped cream.

If you're doing the cooking, fix a meal that you particularly like even if it isn't one of the patient's favorites. (Common sense here, of course: don't give the patient something that a sensitive system can't tolerate.) Make yourself a side dish to balance out something your loved one adores that you consider barely edible.

Always reward yourself for service above and beyond, and be generous about what that means. You don't have to repaint the hallway, but if the dust bunnies are starting to reproduce, give it a good sweep and yourself a treat.

LOCATION, LOCATION, LOCATION

Most self-care advice applies to anybody immersed in caregiving, but some situations call for special responses. One of the biggest of these is where you live physically vis-à-vis the patient.

When You Live There

If you were living with the patient when the medical adventure began, then you probably also have your own local support system. Be sure to keep plugged into that and let your friends help you escape, however briefly.

They may do this by going with you for a meal, a drink, or a movie that isn't on somebody's tablet. A massage, mani-pedi, or walk in the park. Maybe just hanging out and talking the way you always do.

Try to limit discussion of your caregiving or you'll find yourself right back in the middle of what you need to momentarily escape.

You probably know the geographical area well, which gives you a good fix on where to escape for the maximum restoration given the minimum time. Minimum time may be all you have.

You may also ask your local friends to sit in with the patient while you go somewhere all by your lonesome. And don't be in a hurry to come back when you do it.

If you normally live somewhere else but are staying with a parent or other relative during the health crisis, take your local bearings. Get to know neighbors if possible and find the local parks as well as the grocery and pharmacy.

If you grew up here, are old friends still in the area?

In all cases where you are living with the patient, make sure that you get outside the house *every single day* for at least a few minutes. Even if you're standing just outside the door or on the fire escape. You need this release and interaction with the outside world, even if it's ten below zero or ninety-seven in the shade.

It might even be absolutely perfect. Which you won't realize if you don't get out there.

When You Live Somewhere Else

If you're caring for somebody, but not living with them, you have the gift of occasional freedom, taking care of *yourself* on your own terms in your own world.

Yes, you are deeply concerned. Yes, you wish you could do more and you recognize that the road ahead may be rough. But you also have your own life waiting patiently. There's no need to ignore your own life and world or not to enjoy it.

Train yourself to release your concern and anxieties when your caregiving chores end for the day, or when you go home for the weekend. Obsessing and worrying all the time won't help your loved one and it certainly won't help you.

One effective technique is to establish a ritual to transition from the world of your loved one to your own world.

Keep the keys to your dad's apartment in a special bowl reserved just for them or have a jacket that you only wear for caregiving responsibilities. When you get home and put the keys in the bowl or the coat in the closet, stop for a moment. Remind yourself that you are putting away your caregiver responsibilities for now. Send positive thoughts or prayers in whatever fashion you are comfortable with.

Then take a deep breath and step back into your own life.

When You're *Way* Far Away

Whether you're fifty miles away or five hundred, you are a distance caregiver if you can't get to your loved one quickly in case of an emergency.

Learn to decompress consciously on your way home—with a splurge beverage on the plane or special heading-home music you always play in the car.

At home, consolidate caregiving chores (bill paying, following up on stuff, making arrangements) into designated time periods. If you know that Tuesday morning or Wednesday night is when you deal with such-and-such, you give yourself permission not to think about such-and-such at other times.

It's scheduled. You're on it.

If you've assumed responsibility for speaking regularly with your loved one, be particularly careful to schedule that. Make it a convenient time for you, such as on your way to work (hands-free, please), or on your afternoon break (when time is limited!), when you're kicking back as you get home from the office, or on Saturday afternoon when the kids or grandkids are visiting.

Use Zoom or FaceTime for some of your interactions so you can keep track of how the patient looks and acts, as well as how they claim to feel.

SPECIFICS OF SELF-CARE

Get some help.

People get into caregiving ruts and can forget that there are other options. You don't *have* to do everything yourself, and there is nothing particularly attractive about martyrdom.

Talk to your own close friends or to people you know (or can connect with) who have been through similar experiences. Ask them what they did.

Talk to your own doctor if you're having trouble with sleep or anxiety. You may benefit from talk therapy or a short-term course of medication to get you through this rough patch.

Find a support group, either in person or online, if you haven't done so already.

Is housekeeping an issue? Enlist relatives or friends to give the place a thorough once-over and see if they'll commit to follow up on a regular basis. If that isn't an option and you can afford it, hire a cleaning service or housekeeper. A single deep cleaning could hold you for a while and limit disruption.

Hate grocery shopping? We learned during the pandemic that many options for obtaining groceries don't involve pushing your own cart. If these are too expensive, then keep a list and plan the next week's menus to limit your grocery trips.

Always behind on laundry? Try setting up a regular schedule and only do it once a week. Pick a day that isn't normally packed full of other obligations. Start early enough so that you aren't still folding socks at dinner time. Getting everything folded and put away provides more of a psychological boost than you may realize if this isn't your customary M.O.

Expand the Caregiving Circle

How would *you* like to get a break and leave the house for a couple of hours knowing that your responsibilities are covered? Can you arrange to have somebody trustworthy help out during that period? Even better, can you make it a weekly break?

How do you recruit that help without forming an HR department?

Paid assistance may be necessary at any stage of the caregiving process, of course (*see* CHAPTER EIGHT: THE NEW NORMAL).

Volunteer help, however, may be as near as your phone or your own family tree.

In the flurry of activity that begins most caregiving situations, people pop up all the time offering to help, saying: "Just let me know what I can do." Mostly they have no idea what they actually could do but know it's the right thing to say. Maybe they meant to call a week later and ask again, but it kind of slipped their minds.

Now the dust has settled, perhaps literally.

The relatives who came in hurriedly from afar are back home. The neighbors who offered help may be mowing the lawn, but you only see them for a casual wave. Extended family members who were problematic are likely to still be problematic, only now you feel more annoyed than resigned.

So, let's take a look at where you stand.

Pull out that contacts bin you set up when you were collecting business cards at the beginning (*see* CHAPTER TWO: GETTING ORGANIZED). Separate out the medical people and search the cards or scraps of paper for friends and relatives and acquaintances. Now is when it pays off that you noted that that one woman from church is also a quilting friend or that the neighbor on the corner is a handyman. Maybe that woman can do a little hand sewing by her friend's bedside while you catch a matinee. Maybe the handyman can fix the gate that will only close if you push it a certain way.

Seasonal chores? Maybe the youth group from church can rake leaves or a relative's Scout troop can put up storm windows. Perhaps you can get into the knitting circle's Christmas cookie exchange without having to bake anything. If you offer to pay the guy down the block who purely loves riding his snowblower, he may be insulted or he may accept the cash—but either way you're covered when it snows.

Relatives who don't live in town may be willing to come for a week or a weekend and stay with the patient while you take a brief vacation or simply catch up on your sleep and reading. Don't be afraid to ask. Either they'll say yes, or offer an alternate plan, or say no and feel guilty about it.

All of these count as wins for you.

Comfort Yourself

Start with comfort food.

Everybody has favorites. Whether yours is chicken soup or rice pudding or tofu stir-fry or pepperoni pizza—indulge. If you love beef stew and the patient hates it, give them something else and ration your own over several days. And make or buy more than a single serving because you deserve it.

Buy or pick some flowers and put them somewhere other than the sickroom. They're cheap and readily available at grocery stores. If you feel guilty about indulging yourself, get a second bouquet for the patient.

Watch your favorite TV shows or carve out time to binge-watch something you've previously loved or always wanted to find time for.

Avoid Stressful Situations

Yes, that may sound silly. You are living in the center of an extremely stressful situation, or you wouldn't be looking for ways to feel better.

But if current events trouble you, turn off cable news for a few days. It will still be there—probably discussing the same topics—whenever you return. Give yourself a weekend free of social media. Line the birdcage with the newspaper before you read it, rather than after.

If somebody involved in your caregiving group has political views that make you want to scream, ask them very nicely to lay off for now. If asking nicely doesn't work, steel yourself to be firm about it. Keep it neutral. *I really don't want to think about that right now* is better than *How can you possibly believe that?*

There's even an upside. This can be a useful time to jettison activities or responsibilities that are well-established but no longer giving you pleasure or satisfaction. It's hard to argue with somebody who says they need to give up something because they are up to their eyeballs in medical appointments and unexpected responsibilities.

You may promise to try to come back later, but you're under no obligation to do so.

Don't Beat Yourself Up

At every stage of every health crisis, choices are made. Sometimes they're obvious and sometimes you might as well use a dart board.

The critical thing here is to keep looking forward.

Hindsight doesn't help if it upsets you, and most of the time small errors or problems don't matter. Nobody's perfect and we all make mistakes.

Mistakes made out of love can almost always be corrected. And if that isn't possible, a sincere apology is all that's necessary, along with a big smile and a promise to do better.

What is your loved one going to do, anyway? Fire you?

Exercise

If exercise isn't already a part of your own routines, this probably isn't the time to join a gym and hire a personal trainer. Or maybe it's exactly the right time. You can get out, give your body something to do, and maybe even take your mind off Topic A for a little while.

If you already have a solid exercise routine, congratulations. Keep it up.

There may be a piece of unused exercise equipment on a porch or in the basement corner. Remove all the stuff that's piled on it and take it for a little spin.

At the very least take a brief daily walk. It *will* make you feel better, and after a few days, you may find yourself looking forward to it.

Respite Care

Respite care can be formal or informal.

It may be as basic as recruiting another member of the caregiving team (or a relative who lives reasonably nearby) to come spend the weekend while you go home and crash.

Respite care may also be deliciously complex.

Many assisted living and skilled nursing facilities offer the option of having your loved one spend a week or more there while you take off for Tijuana or Tahiti. The quality of this care is likely to be quite good, since lingering in the background is the possibility that you and your loved one will be back later on a more permanent basis.

Find Places to Scream

There will be times in your caregiving experience when you want to scream.

Do yourself a favor before it becomes an emergency: Figure out some places where you can easily and plausibly scream, and don't feel guilty about it for a second.

- Horror movies, especially if you like them anyway.
- Amusement park rides. Here they *want* you to scream. Nor does it need to be a ride where you lose your lunch as well as your inhibitions. A merry-go-round is fine.
- In your car, when you're alone. Don't do this in quiet areas where you might alarm pedestrians or other drivers. Highways are nice if they're not too busy.
- Into a pillow. Take it into the farthest reach of the house, or the garage, or the backyard. Smash your face down into it and let 'er rip.

Burnout

Nobody likes to admit that they feel burned out by caring for a loved one. That just sounds terrible. What do you *mean* that you can't care for your sainted mother? Your beloved spouse? Your favorite sibling? The person who has done so much for you and given you so much for so long?

It's a fact of life, however, and the more you ignore it, the worse it is likely to get.

Caregiving is difficult work with very limited positive feedback.

Burnout is real.

People in your other, previous life won't necessarily want to talk about what you're going through. Sometimes this is through fear that they're likely to wind up in a similar leaky boat before much longer, when one of their own takes a turn.

But here's the thing. You probably *do* know people who've been in a situation similar to your own, even though you may not have discussed it much. They may have even reached out tentatively in the beginning when you were super busy. They're still around, and they haven't forgotten what it's like.

Men are sometimes challenged by this sort of discussion or by sharing personal information. Well, it *is* terribly personal, but so what? You're sharing concerns with a friend, not renting a billboard.

So, talk to people.

Talk to your friends. Talk to the other relatives. Share your feelings, concerns, and anxieties.

Let them remind you that you're doing a great job. Because you undoubtedly are.

Remember that support group you were told about but didn't have time to look into back then? Now may be just the right time to check it out. Finding any kind of emotional support is hugely helpful, whether it's a regular meeting organized by the Alzheimer's Association or an evening with an old friend.

Clergy are trained to counsel and comfort. A visit to or from your own clergyperson (or the patient's) can bring solace and support that you really need right now.

Peek at the Future

Finally, start thinking—just hypothetically, of course—about what the next stage of your caregiving journey might look like and where it might lead. This can be uncomfortable because it brings up a whole range of emotional, financial, and family issues that nobody wants to think about right now (or ever).

Opening the window to the potential next stages may be too painful at the moment, but let the thought flutter through your mind if it wants to. You can close the window again right away if you just can't confront this now.

But don't lock it.

THE FIVE STAGES OF GRIEF

Elisabeth Kübler Ross revolutionized the way people view mourning after death with her Five Stages of Grief.

The same Five Stages can and should be applied to the process of caregiving for serious illness or injury. Keep in mind, however, that these five stages are fluid and don't necessarily adhere to a tidy linear order. You may move back and forth from one to another repeatedly, have several going on at once, or become mired in one section indefinitely. Some stages may not happen at all.

Recognizing where you are in this process can help.

Denial

This one is easy and likely to pop up at regular intervals. Simply stated, you just can't accept that this is happening. It will be over tomorrow or next week or … well, sometime. Maybe down the road a way, but it's going away and then everything will be back to normal, or what seemed like normal before your world blew up.

Denial comes into play with almost every difficult new revelation or situation: A test that reveals what you hoped it wouldn't. A recommendation for treatment that seems too awful to be real. Future plans now shattered in a hundred different ways.

A bad prognosis, of course, can lead to the strongest denial of all.

Anger

This one is also obvious and can run concurrently with any other stage. Physical activity for the caregiver can help with this stage, but however you approach it, getting over anger is generally a very good idea. Not everybody has a punching bag in the basement, or even a basement, though pillows are readily available and very punchable.

Medical folks prefer that you and your loved one get out of the anger stage as quickly as possible. Anger sets off other bodily reactions that generally don't do anyone much good: high blood pressure, distraction, inability to focus, overeating, appetite loss, headaches, difficulty sleeping, tension.

Work on countermeasures to control your own anger: deep breathing, meditation, yoga, long walks, short walks, prayer. Try whatever you have learned over time that can calm you down. If one thing doesn't work, try something else.

When in doubt, take five deep breaths with your eyes closed. It almost always helps and it doesn't use up much time at all.

If you are someone who angers easily, you've probably already heard suggestions about changing that behavior. Maybe you've discussed it with a friend or family member. The bottom line is that you are probably self-aware enough to recognize the problem. Acknowledge it now and take steps to fix or improve it however best you can.

If the patient is the one mired in the quicksand of anger, seek out activities appropriate to somebody in weakened physical condition. Even something as simple as deep breathing *together* with the patient can serve to rearrange emotional reactions.

Bargaining

Bargaining is just what it sounds like. *If my loved one can just get through this test/operation/treatment/illness, I will (fill in your own blank here).*

Bargaining can lead you into strange territory. *I'll give up such-and-such. I won't ever again do this-or-that. I'll be a better person, appreciate my loved one more, learn to be less (or more) self-centered/emotional/rigid/available/demanding/helpful around the house.* These are all noble goals, and maybe you'll follow through on some of them. For the moment, however, it's probably more useful and important to keep putting one foot in front of the other.

Sometimes there isn't much to bargain with or about. In that case, move on.

Depression

Depression is universal and unavoidable at various stages of caregiving.

This is separate and apart from clinical depression that falls into the mental health category. It's being bummed out by what is happening and your inability to fix everything that's gone wrong and facing that you are suddenly on an entirely different road from where you thought you'd be right now.

If you are already under treatment for depression, be sure to stay on your own meds and talk to your psychologist or psychiatrist about what's happening in your life. Your goal is to remain sufficiently functional to carry on, even during your low points.

The same suggestions for dealing with anger can help with depression.

Sleeping more than usual is not uncommon, but after a period of this, you should bring yourself back to your own new reality, however best you can. You've got too many responsibilities to spend half the day with the pillow over your head.

Crawl out of bed and brew some coffee or steep a pot of tea. Walk around the block, or at least to the corner. Do the best you can to keep going.

If you are a Pollyanna by nature, depression may come as something of a shock. Try to roll with it and don't feel that you're any kind of failure for not remaining cheerful. You'll get that cheerful grin back, honest.

Acceptance

Acceptance is generally considered the goal in the traditional Five Stages progression, but it can be the most difficult stage of all.

When you accept your loved one's illness, future, and prognosis—and how these all fit into your own life—you are acknowledging that *maybe* you can't change things. That *probably* you can't change things.

And, finally, that you just plain *can't* change things.

EIGHT
THE NEW NORMAL

M ost caregiving situations start with a flurry of activity. There's so much to be done, and so little time, and so many unanswered questions.

Eventually, however, you begin to realize—and hopefully accept—that you have moved out of crisis mode into your new normal. What's more, everybody in your loved one's family and larger world will also need to accept and adjust to this realization.

Not everybody will reach acceptance at the same time.

This transition isn't easy. In fact, it can be desperately hard. So far, as you struggled and juggled, you were busy reacting. That was the only way to move while hoping things would get better.

Reaction isn't a flaw. It's a reality that allows you to keep trudging forward.

Then one day you begin to accept some combination of these possibilities: (a) the crisis stage has abated, at least for a while; (b) the crisis stage may not conclude in anything resembling the near future; (c) the patient's condition is worsening; and/or (d) the patient either isn't getting better or is doing so at glacial speed.

The world shifts again and slows way down.

MAKE AN ASSESSMENT

You've made earlier assessments of what was happening and where this was likely to lead you. It's time to do the same thing again.

You've learned far more than you realize, education you've absorbed from many directions simultaneously. You may not even remember whose wisdom you have taken to heart and which well-intentioned suggestions you have chosen to ignore.

Take some time now to think about everything. The big picture. The little pictures. The frames of your loved one's life and your own.

There's no rush and there will not be a quiz.

Where Are You Now?

Moving back to the very beginning, consider the patient's initial condition, current condition, and the major intermediary steps. What has been the trajectory? Up, down, sideways? It's likely that you've been on all three paths at one time or another.

Which way is it moving now? Do you anticipate that changing over the next three months? Six months? Year?

What Is the Medical Situation?

This may also have been all over the place, but by now you probably have a pretty clear diagnosis, an established treatment plan, and a pathway for future treatment and medication.

Is this what you were expecting? If not, how does it differ? Are there areas where you anticipate more (or different) treatment in the future?

What Is the Prognosis?

This may or may not be clear. And it may not be good.

If there's a prognosis for a full or significant recovery, you are probably already planning ahead, while perhaps quietly regretting that it's taking so long.

If the prognosis is unclear, why? Is it the nature of the illness, problems particular to this patient, general uncertainty, or a combination of all these factors?

If the prognosis is poor, who made this determination? Medical personnel, the caregiving team, other family and friends, the patient? How has this information affected the patient, family, and caregiving team? Is everyone in agreement with the prognosis?

Are Finances in Order?

At this point, you should be able to snap off a yes or no answer to this one.

If it's yes, congratulations.

If no, consider where you are now and where you were at the beginning. It's quite possible that you've made more progress than you realize. Summarize the remaining liabilities, outstanding obligations, and dangling problems.

Is there something you've put off? Time to get started on it. Take baby steps and begin with something relatively small that you are likely to be able to finish or resolve.

If you've put off seeking professional help until a little bit later—it is now a little bit later.

What's the Living Situation? How Might It Change?

Many long-term caregiving situations will involve changes in environment as matters progress. These issues are pivotal.

These changes may involve physical adaptations to the existing living space, hiring caregiving help, distance care, adult day care, respite care, assisted living, skilled nursing, memory care, and hospice.

If there's no current need to change or adjust the patient's living space, consider yourself fortunate and move on.

What Are Current and Future Caregiving Needs?

This can be difficult to assess or confront, often because nobody really wants to admit that they may have signed on for a lifetime commitment.

Where are you now in terms of time and responsibilities? For your loved one? For yourself? Where are you likely to be down the road a stretch?

Be honest with yourself, even though it may be hard.

If there is a likely or predictable decline in the patient's future, the time to begin thinking about this is now, not when it becomes a sudden crisis and the world blows up again.

After you spend some time with these questions by yourself, you should bring them up with other family members and caregiving teammates. Whether or not they have decision-making authority, you are all in the same boat and the best way to avoid leaks is to make sure it's tightly sealed to begin with.

If you are all geographically convenient to one another, the easiest way to do this is with a relatively informal gathering of the concerned parties. Leave the patient out if you possibly can. Make it a specific meeting with a general agenda and don't spring it on anybody unannounced. Have somebody bring snacks.

If the people involved in these discussions are physically distanced from one another, set something up with Zoom or another online private discussion system. That will allow participants from anywhere on the planet and you'll get to see each other during the discussion.

Taking Away the Keys

This is perhaps the single most-dreaded moment in all caregiving. Losing the ability to get into the car and just go is awful. If you doubt that, take a moment to consider how *you* would manage if you could never drive again.

Enlist the aid of the patient's physician. Sometimes citing "doctor's orders" can help. Or even be enough.

Present a united front with other members of the caregiving team and discuss in advance who will say what. Make sure that your emphasis is on protecting your loved one and keeping them safe, but don't be afraid to use scare tactics if you think they'd be more effective. Even somebody with memory loss understands that you don't want to accidentally plow into a bus stop or wipe out a group of children in a crosswalk.

Be sure to have concrete plans for alternative transportation ready in order to assure your loved one that they will still be able to get around. Insurance sometimes covers transport to medical appointments. Check with the senior center about local shuttle services or with the church for folks to provide grocery shopping transport.

Public transportation can be useful for short hauls if the patient is already comfortable using the system. Uber and Lyft may be problematic, but most areas also have freelance drivers who can be hired for senior transport.

If the vehicle will remain after the patient's driving privileges are gone, put in a kill switch. Or move the car to a different location and say it's in the shop. Substituting keys that won't work on a familiar key ring can also be effective.

Dementia and Memory Impairment

Memory issues in someone you love will break your heart over and over again.

If you are dealing with any form of dementia—or impairment from strokes, traumatic brain injuries, tumors, or seizures, all known as brain "events"—you are far from alone.

That's the good news. The bad news is that most brain events are not reversible. Figuring out how to prevent or fix these problems remains stubbornly elusive. In addition, most forms of dementia grow steadily worse over time.

Invest in the most widely used and respected book, *The 36 Hour Day* by Nancy L. Mace and Peter V. Rabins, now in its sixth edition. Also get the Harvard Medical School Special Reports on *Improving Memory* and *A Guide to Alzheimer's Disease.*

Explore the Alzheimer's Association at *alz.org*, which offers a wide range of publications, seminars, support groups, local resources, and information for caregivers—along with a 24/7 helpline at 800-272-3900. This is an excellent way to find a support group, and you should have one.

The Family Caregiver Alliance (*caregiver.org*) has many related publications, including the excellent *Caregiver's Guide to Understanding Dementia Behaviors.*

The unfortunate reality of dementia caregiving is that when you are in the thick of it, there usually is little time for any of this. In addition, because your loved one looks the same and may cycle in and out of dementia behaviors, outsiders can be judgmental if you're having trouble dealing with it.

Be very careful to take care of your own health and emotional well-being. Self-care is essential for your survival, since with dementia, the patient will grow increasingly unaware of your needs.

Remind yourself regularly that you are doing the best you can for both of you.

Safety

A primary consideration in care for the memory-impaired is the patient's safety.

You must take basic steps to guard their safety and physical well-being. These will vary from one situation to another, but all require vigilance.

A major consideration is whether your loved one is living alone, or with you, or with somebody else who may not be up to the required responsibilities.

If you are living together, you know what happens when and you know where the weak points are. Otherwise, you need to observe on the scene, preferably for at least twenty-four hours.

Don't make assumptions based on past behavior, no matter how regular that may have been. A former early bird may be watching television at midnight eating oatmeal.

Expect the patient to deny problems, argue against precautionary steps, and pull out their "A" game for medical personnel. Personal awareness of what's happening to someone can foster creative ways to hide problems because—in their more lucid moments—they know exactly what is happening and fear the unnamed future even more than you do.

The Safety Survey

Conduct a safety survey of your loved one's living space and observe issues that are likely to cause problems. Try to find short-term solutions if possible, because in this dreadful game of whack-a-mole, new challenges appear regularly.

Pay particular attention to kitchens, basements, work rooms, and outdoor areas. Are there power tools and equipment that can create problems? Chemicals or caustic materials? Guns or other weapons? These all have the potential to cause major problems and should be put away, removed, or locked up.

If your loved one turns on the stove and wanders away, or shows other carelessness in the kitchen, you can remove burner knobs or install hidden valves or switches for turning on cooktops. Move potentially dangerous kitchen tools to a higher location or off-site. Keep electrical appliances away from water and the sink. Many electrical kitchen items come with automatic shut-off features.

While we're in the kitchen: food spoils. Keep an eye on foodstuffs left overnight on the counter or held far past their expiration dates. Clear the fridge routinely of potential sources of food poisoning.

Keep medications locked up.

Check all the existing safety equipment to be sure it is up to date and has fresh batteries. A smoke detector that's dead or an ancient fire extinguisher is a tremendous hazard.

The Wanderer

Wandering off is a major issue for some patients and is often how faraway relatives first become aware of dementia issues.

If you live with the wanderer, you may be able to simply add latches or door locks that aren't at eye level. A high or low bolt on outside doors may be all you need. Doorknobs can be removed. Consider an electronic locking system. Any time the patient is locked in, of course, an adult must be on the premises in case of fire.

Put a spare house key in a convenient location near the door for accidental lockouts and leave another with a neighbor if possible. Ask that same neighbor and others in the area to keep an eye out and notify you if your loved one manages to slip away.

Finding the Lost

Medical alert jewelry is critical (*see* CHAPTER SIX: THE DAILINESS OF DAILY LIFE).

A memory-impaired patient who wanders off may not remember their name or where they live, but anybody can push the button on Medic-Alert jewelry and call for help.

The Alzheimer's Association has a joint (paid) program with Medic-Alert to help locate and return patients who wander off. You can also locate the cell phone of somebody who carries the appropriate app. GPS-related systems for tracking people are sometimes available.

Organizing for Memory Impairment

When in doubt, don't.

You may think you're doing your loved one a favor by moving things to a location that is more convenient, but most of the time that just makes things inaccessible. Try to keep stuff where the patient has always kept it.

If minor changes are necessary, make every effort to keep things together that are used together. Keys in the same drawer or on the same rack, outdoor clothing on the same hooks or in the same closet, coffee by the coffee maker.

If you move the patient to a new location, however, all bets are off.

Here you can do what makes sense, but you have to figure out ways for your loved one to find what they're looking for. Pictures and/or labels on kitchen cabinets (dishes, glasses, canned goods, spices, pots and pans) are a good start. If that's too complicated, consider taking the cabinet doors off and leaving items in plain sight.

Conversing with Dementia

Of all the frustrations in dealing with somebody whose memory no longer works correctly, conversation heads the list. It can also be the most heartbreaking.

Essentially, you need to relearn everything you know about conversation. The Alzheimer's Association has extensive material on this issue.

Speaking louder doesn't help. Repeating something doesn't help. Telling somebody they already know the answer to a question is useless. Correcting misinformation won't work.

Things not to say: "Don't you remember?" "I've told you and told you." "We already discussed this." "Weren't you paying attention?" "How many times do I need to tell you?"

Ask yes-or-no questions or offer specific choices to keep options clear. "Do you want a turkey or ham sandwich?" is better than "What do you want for lunch?"

Take a deep breath, summon any reserves of patience that remain, and answer the patient's question for the four hundredth time. Explain one more time what you're doing or where you're going. Remind your loved one to put their coat on, or take their hat off, or wear their shoes when you go outside.

If they no longer recognize you, or think you're their long-deceased sister, don't try to argue the point. Smile and ask a question about something the two of them might have done back in better days. When old memories are all that remain, they are important.

If your loved one is adamant about something, it may be easier to just agree and change the subject. Creative fibbing is not merely acceptable. Sometimes it's all that stands between you and a long inappropriate scream.

Assistive Devices

"Assistive devices" covers a lot of territory.

Essentially this means any device that makes life easier for the patient and/or caregiver, in either the long or short run. That can range from a long shoehorn to a motorized scooter—with countless intermediate stops. It may include things you've never heard of that are absolutely perfect.

You are probably already using the obvious devices for your situation. Take a look at how and where you're using them. Is there an easier or more efficient way?

Pay particular attention to anything you find annoying.

There's some overlap here with adapting the physical

environment, covered later in this section and focused on the home.

Shelley Peterman Schwarz has written a wonderful book filled with ideas for adapting your living space to your particular needs, on both large and small scales. *Home Accessibility: 300 Tips for Making Life Easier* is an excellent investment. In addition, you should check with your support groups to see what they have found useful (or not).

Voice Activation and Remote Devices

All sorts of technology can be easily and inexpensively adapted to voice commands. Somebody with recently diminished small motor skills may find such systems fantastic or they may hate them. It's usually worth a try.

If small keys are the issue, or the TV remote is so complicated it could run a space shuttle, look into items with bigger buttons and fewer of them.

Robots

There aren't nearly enough of these for common use just yet, but dedicated machinery to clean floors has gone mainstream. These independent vacuum cleaners and floor washers are easy to use, and some are quite inexpensive.

You might also consider Siri and Alexa and the others who do your electronic voice bidding as part of your robotic staff.

Computers and Other Tech Devices

Any time you buy a computer, phone, television or other piece of technology, it is obsolete before you get it in the trunk of your car. So, we'll speak in generalities.

A lot depends on the tech sophistication levels of both user and caregiver.

Somebody who's already had their world turned inside out may not welcome changes to a previously comfortable system. Pushing new tech on someone who isn't interested creates new problems under the guise of fixing old ones.

This is not the time to get your loved one a spiffy new laptop or a fancy new cell phone unless they are totally invested in the idea and willing to learn how to use it.

One possible exception is the tablet, which is lightweight and portable with a touch screen. It's just fine for email, surfing, streaming, and Zoom chats.

There are also ways to make even the most outdated computer system easier for somebody recovering from major health problems. A bigger keyboard, for instance, or a larger monitor. A more comfortable or appropriate desk chair. Your best bet is to Google your general need, such as "computer devices for disabled users." Then follow those responses down any rabbit holes that seem appropriate.

Getting Around

If this is an issue, you are undoubtedly already using some kind of equipment to make locomotion easier. Is it the best solution? Again, these things change frequently.

You should have a disabled parking permit by now. If not, move that to the top of your to-do list and call the doctor's office.

If your loved one is already using a walker or wheelchair, does it have places to store things like glasses or knitting supplies? Is there a cup holder? Google "wheelchair accessories" for lots of other possibilities.

Vehicles for people with major movement problems can be tricky and expensive. Some cars are hard to get in and out of, even for the young and limber. Add years and ailments and it gets a lot harder. You may even need to accept that the vehicle you've been using is no longer appropriate.

Vans for people with disabilities offer all kinds of very specific features, both for driving and for getting people and their major equipment in and out. These vehicles are not cheap, but if you really need one and the patient is willing, don't be too proud to ask for help finding and paying for it. Maybe a wealthy relative can kick in or somebody knows somebody with a connection. If you have access to a local service organization such as Rotary or Kiwanis, perhaps they'll take on the project as a fundraiser. A church may collect contributions or have the youth group sponsor a pancake breakfast.

It is not a weakness to request financial assistance for something major that is necessary after a medical event changes someone's life.

Vision and Hearing Assistance

If vision or hearing assistance is a new and/or major concern, your health care provider has probably already made suggestions or authorized insured items. Be wary, however, if somebody wants to sell you something that your insurance doesn't cover. At least do a little comparison shopping.

Begin with a broad and basic Google search and narrow it down as you consider options. "Vision aids for the disabled" will take you down paths you never realized exist.

And don't forget the obvious. Magnifying glasses have been around a long time and they get the job done.

Hearing issues are problematic in the best of times, since people with diminished hearing may not realize or admit it. Hearing aids also have a deserved reputation for not working the way people want them to.

Medicare doesn't cover hearing aids as a general rule, and they don't come cheap. But some Medicare Advantage or Medicap/Supplemental policies offer partial coverage.

Decide how hard you want to push the hearing aid issue, and if necessary resign yourself to shouting. Wireless earphones for TV or phone calls can help. Closed captioning is available for almost everything, and while it's often a little off (particularly with the news), it can still be very useful.

Reachers

Reachers are wonderful, and people who use them often wonder how they ever managed before. Many folks keep them in several different rooms for different reasons.

Essentially these are arm extenders with rubberized gripping claws at the end for items on top shelves or in low corners. They're a fine substitute for a stepstool, particularly if climbing is no longer wise for the patient. Check out different styles and lengths to see what works best for you.

Make sure you practice with the patient. And don't use a reacher to get down breakable items. Move those to a lower shelf.

Reachers are versatile, but they don't clean up broken glass.

Air Quality

A patient with respiratory issues needs to be in an environment that is clean and free of dust and pollutants.

If the patient's living space seriously needs cleaning and you haven't quite gotten around to it, now is the time. Hire help if you can afford it. Or enlist help wherever you can find and try to make it a good-natured project with lots of pizza.

For a patient in an area with poor outside air quality, keep the windows closed and have any duct systems cleaned so you don't keep recirculating the same grime. Put an air cleaner in the bedroom and another wherever your loved one spends a lot of time.

Change filters regularly on anything that has them: furnace, A/C, ceiling vent, vacuum, air cleaner.

Service Animals

Trained service dogs go through years of specialized training, mostly from volunteers, before being permanently assigned to people who require their help to remain independent. Their skills are customized to the owner's needs.

When a service dog is with their person, you should barely be aware of their presence.

These animals do not sniff crotches, pee inappropriately, bark at other dogs, jump around, or play with children. Their job is to help one person, and that's what they do.

There is no official certification or vest for a legitimate service animal, though a plentitude of both can be purchased online, including for purse dogs. Only dogs or miniature horses (yes, really) are officially recognized by the American Disability Act (ADA) as trained service animals. However, establishments are very limited by ADA regulations about questioning the validity of alleged service animals.

A gray area of "emotional support animals" has grown, and many people are legitimately dependent upon them. However, pigs, ducks, monkeys, peacocks, gliding possums, and snakes are no longer allowed on airplanes as emotional support animals.

If your loved one could benefit from the use of a service dog, start investigating options as early as possible. There's almost always a lot of time and paperwork involved. And there are never enough trained service animals to go around.

Clothing

Adaptive-design clothing can be easily put on and removed, a blessing for anyone who no longer has the dexterity to handle back fasteners, tiny buttons, hooks, and snaps.

Front-closure clothing is useful for the ambulatory as well. Many items are also specifically designed for people who use wheelchairs, with a solid front and Velcro at the back.

Velcro can be your new best friend, holding together jackets, sweaters, skirts, and pants.

Shoes with Velcro and a long shoehorn can also make footwear manageable again.

Adapting the Physical Environment

You've probably been doing this already, often without realizing it. Changes tend to be gradual and reactive.

Now is the time to codify those "temporary" changes and to see what else can be done to make home life more efficient.

Stop procrastinating. It's time to deal with whatever changes you've put off.

Fresh eyes can help a lot. If you know someone with an eye for efficient design or a knack for problem-solving and organizing, ask or hire that person to help. Explain your particular needs (wheelchair access, staircases, kitchen management, lighting) and then show them the specifics you'd like to improve or modify.

If you're working with a physical therapist or occupational therapist, get their input on adaptations to make life easier, both now and down the line.

The patient may dislike, resent, or object to these changes. If you feel they're necessary, stand your ground and promise they're only temporary. Cross your fingers if you know that's not quite true and smile while you do it.

Major exception: If dementia is an issue, avoid moving things around. Anywhere. If you absolutely must move things, provide obvious labels or pictures to show the patient where they are.

Outside

How does your loved one get into the house or apartment?

An elevator? Stairs? Even one or two stairs can be a problem for somebody with mobility issues. If there aren't already outdoor stair railings, install them or speak to the landlord. Older people in general become more dependent on railing, so this may also benefit you.

Is entry through a garage or mud room or side door that everybody always uses? Make sure any obstacles are long gone from these pathways and that there's a place to sit and remove boots.

If you've been pretending that you won't need a ramp and it's now pretty obvious that you do, follow local code specifications and make sure the work is done by somebody who knows what they're doing. You need railings here, too, and you can't skimp on this one.

Are outside pathways clear and even? Broken concrete or other uneven surfaces can create major havoc from tiny stumbles.

If there's a patio or backyard, can your loved one get out and enjoy it? This may be as simple as rearranging outdoor furniture or moving the barbecue grill or it may require adding another railing or two.

If your loved one is a gardener, they may already have a head start, using things like a kneeler/seat, raised beds, long-handled tools, and a garden toolbelt with plenty of pockets. If mobility is a new issue, the gardener can probably help figure out adaptations.

However, if the yard has always been a mess and your loved one ignores it anyway, don't bother. Just have it periodically mowed or scythed.

Outside lighting is critical, particularly if anyone ever arrives after dark. (This includes paramedics.) You definitely need a light shining on the street number, which should also be shown clearly at the curb. Solar lights along a pathway are cheap and very helpful, as are motion-activated outdoor lights, whether hardwired, plugged into weatherproof outlets, or battery-operated. Position these closer together than you think you need to.

If your loved one lives alone and may need to call 911, get a lockbox so EMTs can enter without breaking windows. Check with local authorities to see what they prefer.

Stairs

Two-story residences provide specific challenges. So do basements. You may already have dealt with some of them, perhaps by temporarily relocating the patient to the ground floor.

Maybe that first-floor space needs to be made a bit more finished and permanent, in a modified "bedroom." You might even swap out some of the actual bedroom furniture. Add a nice screen or two for privacy.

If vision is a bigger problem than climbing stairs, you can paint the stair risers a contrasting color. Even easier, put a strip of colored painter's tape on the edge of each step. Motion-activated strip lights also work well.

If funds permit, consider adding a seat that travels up and down the staircase. If funds *and* space permit, you might even tuck in a little elevator.

All stairways should have bannisters or railings on both sides.

This usually isn't too difficult between first and second stories, but basements often are unfinished or slapdash. If there's any chance that the patient is going to go down there for any reason, you need a railing. Try to also provide lighting that doesn't require reaching out to grab a doohickey on the end of a dangling string.

Hallways and Doorways

Clear hallways as much as possible, removing throw rugs and unnecessary furniture. All furniture, if possible. A patient using a wheelchair or scooter needs lots of space to navigate and turn. You may also need room to hover or walk beside someone using a cane or a walker.

If doorways are tight or problematic, remove the doors by the hinges. Doorstops can be elegant or inexpensive, so long as they keep the door open. Various attachments can simplify opening doorknobs or levers.

Doorways leading to the outdoors often have a slight step up. Rubber threshold slopes are available commercially at a very specific range of heights to offer an unbroken surface.

If there are places that you *don't* want the patient to go, particularly with dementia, consider a hook or simple sliding lock way up high or way down low where it's not obvious.

Sickroom/Bedroom

The sickroom was once known as the bedroom, and as much as possible, you should try to return it to that incarnation.

By now you may have adjusted or replaced the bed, adding tray tables, guard rails, and/or a commode. If you've added hospital furniture, look for ways to soften the stark feeling, starting with a nice looking bedspread or quilt. Add a potted plant or silk roses, and make sure there's a good reading lamp that the patient can easily turn on.

For somebody who isn't supposed to get out of bed without help—but does!—look into bedside mats that sound an alarm when they're stepped on.

Before we leave the bedroom, take a look at your loved one's clothing and where it's stored. When a patient begins to get dressed in something other than pajamas or sweats, they are likely to be using a different and more limited wardrobe than their previous one. Consider what your loved one is actually wearing now and making some minor storage adjustments.

You don't need to declutter clothing just now and shouldn't even think about it unless your loved one makes the suggestion. However, you can group their current favorite items in the same easily accessed part of the closet and put frequently worn things in a couple of convenient dresser drawers. Don't forget shoes, socks, and underwear.

Once again, promise that this is "just temporary," because maybe it is.

Bathroom

Bathrooms take up less space with more potential for problems than any other room.

Start with everything being hard and designed to not absorb water. Add water from multiple locations.

Factor in excretion, which people need to do easily and routinely.

Hand and body washing requires faucets and a bathtub or shower stall. To bathe you need to take off all your clothes in a small space, get in and out of the shower or tub, then dry off and dress. Most people also shampoo in the shower.

Many people take their routine medications in the bathroom and may keep a scale in there for when the clothes are off. Those who wear makeup are likely to apply it in the bathroom, and we all know where everybody is supposed to brush and floss multiple times a day.

For anyone over the age of fifty—or *any* age if falling is an issue or likely to become one—you need grab bars in multiple locations. Start on the inside tub or shower wall, with a second bar outside where you step in. You may also want one by the toilet.

You *must* use grab bars that screw into the wall, since even the best stick-ons may fail when yanked hard and fast. Have them professionally installed so you're sure they can take the full weight of someone who's about to crash.

A seat or stool inside the shower or outside the tub permits safer bathing. Hand-held shower attachments make it easy to get clean all over. Soap on a rope can't be dropped.

Keep all items used in the shower or tub together, on an accessible shelf or in a waterproof container with a handle and holes in the bottom. Bathtubs should have rubber mats with suction cups, sandpapery stick-ons, or both.

Walk-in bathtubs are expensive but safe and comfortable for those who love to soak but can't easily use a conventional bathtub.

Toilet modifiers have lots of different configurations, starting with handrails and raised seats, then moving through built-ins or add-ons such as bidet attachments.

Sharp edges and corners can be made safer with the soft pads sold to babyproof furniture.

Get rid of any bath rugs that are not anchored firmly. It's nice to have something warm under your bare feet, but it isn't worth taking a tumble. If you must have something, look for rugs with thick rubber bases that hug the floor energetically.

Remove anything that doesn't need to be readily accessible, like a giant stack of towels or nine rolls of toilet paper in a cute holder. You may need to move other things in, such as an adult diaper disposal unit.

Clear the shower and tub of any extra, empty, or disappointing products. All you need to keep out are the current soap, shampoo, and conditioner. Do the same thing around the sink, where odd jars and bottles tend to congregate and breed.

Think about what your loved one does in the bathroom. Where should the equipment and materials be for easiest access? Hairbrushes, hairdryers, oral hygiene materials, and shaving equipment can all live on the vanity if there's room.

You may want a stool for makeup and hair drying. Separate out the most frequently used makeup items and put them in a small basket on the counter, perhaps beside a new and easily adjusted makeup mirror.

Meds should be in a dispenser on the counter, in the top drawer, or on the bedside table.

Are light switches at an easy level? Can the door be propped open for easier access?

Make sure there's a nightlight inside the bathroom and another outside the entry, whether that's in the bedroom or the hall. Get the kind that light up when it's dark, so you won't need to think about them again till they burn out.

The Home Office

Whether it's a dedicated room with a door that closes or a nook in the bedroom, kitchen, or family room, somebody has undoubtedly been using the home office as the health crisis evolved. Quite possibly, it's you. So, you already know any flaws that may exist. Fix them unless your loved one is likely to reclaim that space soon.

If a dedicated home office is upstairs but your loved one comes down only once and stays all day, relocate the office to the first floor. The dining table makes a dandy home office.

Kitchen

For some people, the only silver lining to being ill or incapacitated is not having to cook. That person's kitchen can be set up to accommodate caregivers and visitors. Want the coffeemaker in a different spot? Just move it.

Folks who enjoy cooking and have done a lot of it, however, may need more serious adjustments. A padded floor mat can make standing more comfortable. Perhaps your loved one would be happier working while seated at a stool by the counter or on a rolling chair at the table.

Soft-handled tools are easier to hold. Jar openers, cookbook stands, and electric can openers can all be mounted on walls. Move anything previously reached by stepstool to a lower level.

Work with an enthusiastic cook to determine what equipment they use most often, then gather those things in a convenient location. Favorite pans can reside on top of the stove. Keep favorite bowls, knives, utensils, measuring implements, dishes, glasses, and flatware in a single, easily accessed spot. Frequently used cookbooks, ingredients, and seasonings should also be clustered together. A rolling cart can work well for this if there's room.

Don't try to talk the cook into thinning out an excess of sauté pans or anything else. Leave things that aren't used often in place unless you need that shelf or drawer for the regularly used items.

MOVING ON

Time brings change.

At some point, you're probably going to need more help.

Usually the steps here are incremental, both heading into the situation and moving through it. This process sometimes also begins with an event that drops you smack into the new phase, ready or not.

Often that event is a fall.

Some of the following options may have been a part of the patient's care in earlier stages, and it can feel like a reversal to need them again. Try to regard this new process as helping retain control for both patient and caregiver.

Even if there's a specific reason why now is the time, expect resistance from the patient. Brace yourself for firm denial or outright hostility.

Loss of independence is difficult. You may need to slide into this subject gently and hypothetically at first, and that still may not help. Present a united front with the others involved in your loved one's caregiving if at all possible. It's harder to fight everybody.

Almost all options from here on out come at a price, both emotional and financial.

Long-Term Care Insurance

If the patient already has long-term care insurance, you are way ahead of the game. By the time you need it in most caregiving situations, it is far too late to apply or be approved.

Qualifying to use it and actually getting paid, however, can be problematic. Figure out exactly how the policy works and what is and isn't covered. Ask plenty of questions. Prepare for mountains of paperwork.

In some cases, a family member may qualify for payment, but don't count on that until you have it verified in writing. And don't spend a nickel until the insurance check clears.

Adult Day Care

You may be able to hold off on making major care changes for a while if there are options for adult day care in your area.

Essentially this is a scheduled time where your loved one goes to another location to spend time with others at similar levels of illness or disability. There may be a meal involved, and there will almost certainly be available activities.

For folks who've always had a social orientation, this can be a fabulous opportunity. For the more private and withdrawn it may not work at all.

It will accomplish two things, however. First, it will give you a regular break, even if there's barely enough time between drop-off and pickup to stare at the wall for half an hour in peace. Second, this transitional stage can accustom your loved one to being around new people in a different location, which will be useful when it's time to consider assisted living.

Local Check-In Services

Some communities offer a check-in service for seniors through the senior center or police department. Volunteers make daily calls to seniors living alone to see how they're doing and notice if something sounds amiss. Then once a week, somebody comes by and visits in person. You are their contact if they notice problems.

Paid Check-In Services

These are the same concept, at a price.

Some of these are mechanized and require only that your loved one pick up the phone and say hello. Others have a real person on the other end.

If there's no answer, or somebody sounds disoriented or un-
like their previous self, these services will notify 911 and you as
the contact person.

Meals on Wheels

Meals on Wheels takes the check-in concept one important step
further, providing food and nutrition on a daily basis, by delivery
or in group settings such as senior centers. The program goal is
that no older person should go hungry for lack of funds or the
ability to prepare food.

If your loved one is living alone and cooking has become
a problem, Meals on Wheels can be a nutritional lifesaver and
also prolong independent living. Delivery volunteers become a
personal connection, as well as a conduit to alert you and local
EMTs or health agencies should new problems arise.

Meals on Wheels is available all over the country, though
some areas with more need than funding may have wait lists.
Individuals pay on a sliding scale based on need, from nothing
to full price. Check what's available in your location by visiting
mealsonwheelsamerica.org.

Family Moving In

At some point, check-in services and meal delivery may not
be enough.

If the patient has been living alone, or you're the only live-in
caregiver, one useful intermediate step is to have a family mem-

ber or very close friend come and stay for a while as you work out this new stage.

Unless you have family members with great dedication and flexibility, this period isn't likely to last long. But it can buy some time. It's even possible that the newcomer will like this new location and its amenities and want to stick around.

It's usually less expensive to work with family, because they feel stronger obligations, but don't try to totally cheap it out. Room and board is nice, but if the room is an army cot in the basement and the board is a pantry full of Ensure, you need to sweeten the pot.

Bringing in Outside Help

Perhaps you had outside help in the early stages of caregiving, during the initial period when specialized assistance is necessary after hospitalization. In that high-pressure time, decision-making is often rushed and the big picture blurry at best.

The good news is that now you probably have more time to figure out what you want and need to do. The even better news is that you are much more familiar with the ins and outs of caregiving in general and your loved one's situation in particular.

Unless there's a major precipitating emergency, it's best to start by bringing in help for limited periods. This helps everybody get used to the new situation and is considerably less expensive.

Government Assistance

Your loved one may be eligible for government assistance,

which varies from one state to another and also sometimes by county or town. Eligibility is usually based on need and determined by a social worker assessment. It takes a while to set up.

Check with local authorities to see if this is a possibility. Contact the doctor's office or call your town or county government office for a referral.

What's covered? That depends. Sometimes it's only medical assistance, or it may include housekeeping and personal care.

You have less control in this situation, and you don't get to decide who comes in to do what, but the price is right. And it can mean the difference between your loved one staying at home or needing to move elsewhere, at least for now.

Hiring Help

Here's everybody's fantasy: A sweet and energetic nursing student needs housing and is willing to work for free to gain experience.

This situation does not exist in real life.

If you need to hire outside help, it can feel overwhelming. It usually *is* overwhelming, so ease into things if you possibly can. Keep in mind that there are never enough top-notch caregivers available. Ever.

Start by asking around.

Check with your local support group for referrals, as well as for people and agencies to avoid. Ask your online support group for guidance on what skills are most important for your specific situation. Do you have friends or fellow church members who've hired outside help? Somebody who knows somebody can be an excellent start.

Agencies are expensive, and a big chunk of what you pay them never reaches the caregiver. If money isn't an issue, however, this may be your best option. The agency will vet employees, refer you to satisfied customers, have replacement or substitute caregivers available, and bear some responsibility if things don't work out.

Ask the agency for references, check those references thoroughly, and read any contract carefully before you sign. Learn in advance how either side may end the arrangement. This is much easier when you're all still good buddies.

If your loved one lives in a senior community, you may be able to piggyback on a neighbor with a part-time employee. But don't poach. Check first with whoever is paying the bills about costs, qualifications, responsibilities, and availability.

If you are placing or responding to an ad online or in a local publication, be particularly vigilant about references. Our imperfect world includes crooks who will ignore your loved one and rob them blind, all while exuding competence and charm.

When hiring someone you don't know, be sure to ask their references about problems or concerns. Ask how *they* first came to hire the candidate. Think about what's important in your situation and make a list of questions so you don't forget anything.

Make your questions for the references open-ended but specific: "What do you wish she might have done a little differently?" is more likely to lead into a candid response than "How did you like her?"

Trust your gut on things that just don't seem right, either from references or the candidate. Try not to seem desperate, even if you are.

The devil is in the details, and you need to work them out in advance. Who's going to do the grocery shopping? The cooking? The laundry? Understand that major housekeeping is rarely part of the package.

If transportation of your loved one is necessary for any reason, be sure the caregiver is licensed and insured. This is even more important if they'll be using their own car.

Be around during the transition period and watch carefully. Make it clear that there is a probationary period and set terms. Somebody who seemed perfect may present problems you hadn't considered. Or, if you're lucky, somebody iffy who was the best you could find may turn out to be a jewel.

Don't expect too much from a part-time hired caregiver. Hiring help may lighten your own load, but it won't really solve anything.

If you have more than one caregiving shift, make sure the various employees interact with one another. Instruct them how to debrief at the end of a shift.

Finally, caregiving is notoriously underpaid, but it can still be a real bite.

Moving in with Relatives

This can be very easy or almost impossible.

If there are relatives—nearby or at a distance—who are willing to take in your loved one and have the time, temperament, and space to do so, congratulations.

The wild card here is your loved one, who may be firmly opposed to going anywhere. If that's the case, unless their level of disability is so strong that all other options are worse, you may not be able to carry through on this.

Get tough here if you need to and if the living situation feels promising. Mention that assisted living and nursing homes are alternative solutions, particularly if you know this worries the patient. Present the proposed option as a way to put off those possibilities, at least for now.

A secondary wild card pops up if your loved one agrees. You then need to decide what will happen to the patient's current residence, furniture, and personal effects.

Economics drives this situation.

If money is tight, you probably can't afford to maintain two residences. If the patient is on a downward trajectory or stabilized at a level that requires considerable care, the likelihood of returning to solitary living diminishes.

Closing out a house or apartment is far too complex a topic to tackle here, but if you do need to drastically downsize your loved one's living situation, make sure that the things that ultimately matter don't get lost in the confusion. Hang on to photographs, special pieces of art, a favorite comfortable chair, beloved clothing, the marital bedstead, important books, and … whatever. It's different for everybody but it's always important.

Take pictures of what can't come along, print them, and put them in an album.

Make sure your loved one realizes through all of this that you love them dearly and are as sad as they are that things can't remain the same.

MOVING INTO A FACILITY

This scares almost everybody.

It's the most dramatic possible change, and it answers the question of what will come next with all too much clarity.

Don't put me in a Place.

That's what it all boils down to, and the reality is that you are trying to do precisely that, even if it's breaking your heart.

There's also an awareness of permanency and decline that accompanies this decision. How you handle this and negotiate the next steps is entirely dependent upon who your loved one is and what all of you think is best.

Retirement Communities

Might as well start with the best possible solution.

Most areas have at least one high-end retirement facility built upon this concept: People move in and remain in the community for the rest of their lives, with pleasant surroundings, physical comfort, available medical assistance, and a cohort of like-minded (and like-funded) friends.

If your loved one does not have a healthy retirement fund and additional assets, you can probably skip this section.

Residents buy into this type of facility—with a direct payment, the purchase of a unit, or both. Once in residence, they will almost certainly be charged for meals, whether they eat them or not. (The food is usually excellent.) Activities of all sorts are available, and newcomers may already know other residents.

Residency usually begins with an apartment or cottage.

Should a resident or their spouse begin to have problematic physical or mental issues, that person can move into the assisted living section. Here there's less space but still some independence, with any partner still living right there on the grounds. Extra caregiving help is almost always available at a price, though levels of assistance may vary from one community to another. Outside medical assistance is almost always readily available.

Down the road, should someone's health turn on them—either slowly or dramatically—the on-site nursing home will have a bed. There is probably a memory care unit if needed. Hospice is generally also available on location when it's time.

Throughout it all, residents maintain the same address.

Assisted Living

Assisted living is an intermediate step for people who have been living on their own or with family, but now require more consistently available, hands-on care.

People don't just decide to go into assisted living. They have to qualify.

Need is determined on a state-by-state basis by a formal medical and personal assessment. Prospective residents may present with a wide range of deficits. Some people are unable to move easily but remain very sharp mentally. Others are physically fit with serious mental lapses. Some are a combination. Spouses are usually able to move into the same room even if they don't meet disability criteria.

Since this is always a continuum, any facility has a range of residents. At some point, residents may require more care than is authorized and need to move into a nursing home.

Assisted living expenses may be covered by Medicaid or paid privately. They are generally not cheap.

These facilities usually offer exercise, organized activities, laundry, meals, medication dispensing, transit to medical visits, and camaraderie. Doctors are available and a nurse is on site or on call nearby. Meals are included, and units often have mini fridges for personal favorite foods.

Generally, one can move in their own furniture, a comfortable transition. Residents bring their own TV and electronics. Some places even allow small pets.

Do your research and make exploratory visits without your loved one. Not every place is right for every resident, and somebody who's already reluctant will dig their heels in harder if you drag them to a place that is obviously not right for them.

When you find a place that you think is a good fit, *then* bring them. There are a limited number of rooms, so understand that they may not be able to move in immediately. Sometimes a place will know an opening is coming if somebody is leaving to live with relatives or for extra care in a nursing home.

Ask how often rooms usually become available, though of course this is beyond anybody's control. There may also be a long waiting list of people who have applied but aren't quite ready yet.

When you begin to look into assisted living facilities, start by realistically assessing your loved one and how they are going to fit into this new kind of community.

Someone who's shy or withdrawn benefits from the intimacy and privacy of a smaller place. A more sociable and gregarious person might prefer a larger group of fellow residents.

In either case, pay close attention to the staff and other residents. These will change over time, of course. But if the staff seems rude or unresponsive now, remember that you are still in the courtship stage. It won't get better.

Try to visit during a meal so you can see everybody gathered in one place (and get a look at the food, as well). Do residents and staff seem comfortable with each other? Interact easily? Seem content, if not happy? Are the communal areas comfortable and inviting?

Check the weekly schedule and see what happens on a planned basis. Ask staff and/or residents what they like to do. Clarify how staff coordinates with the patient's current doctors.

Nursing Homes

Nursing homes had an unfortunate reputation long before COVID-19.

Concerns exploded, justifiably, once the pandemic began.

But the thing about nursing homes is that when you need them, you *really* need them. So, let's get general nursing home concerns out of the way first, because when the time comes—and it can happen overnight—there won't be much in the way of alternatives.

People go into nursing homes because they have serious problems, not quite bad enough for hospitalization but way too serious to be at home or in assisted living. As far as Medicare and insurance are concerned, however, they are expected to be transitional.

This creates a lot of secondary problems, mostly versions of *What now?*

Nursing home concerns often center around the help, who are notoriously underpaid and never sufficiently available. Or sufficient, for that matter. There is a perennial shortage of people willing to work for sub-minimum wage in facilities that are not, overall, fun places to be.

People fear having their loved one's possessions stolen, their personal hygiene ignored, their concerns and needs unheeded, their meds forgotten, their bedsores unattended, and so on and so on.

However, when your loved one lands in a nursing home, you probably won't have a lot of notice. It never happens when you're ready. Still, you need to swing into action right away, because various clocks are already ticking, and you need to get things done.

Who's covering what? What do the docs expect to happen next? Are there options?

Medicare limits payment for nursing homes, usually to two weeks. This can be enough for post-op knee replacement, but woefully inadequate for brain events.

Be prepared to give this move a lot of time and attention for a while.

Memory Care Units

This is the hardest one of all.

You are admitting to yourself that your loved one isn't just a little fuzzy, or getting over something, or not quite themselves. They are being called on by the visitor nobody wants to identify out loud, delivering a diagnosis nobody wants to hear.

Most people put off placing family members into memory care for a while after they accept that it's necessary, for all sorts of legitimate reasons. Friends and family won't understand why you can't do it yourself. Your loved one has occasional lucid moments that suggest you've got more time. You promised them in a weak moment that you'd never do it.

Unless there's major antisocial behavior involved, you probably *do* have a bit more time.

But not enough. Time is now your fiercest enemy. You're

watching someone you love as they slide out of awareness of your life together and into a netherworld that you can't enter.

Memory care units are specially designed facilities that approximate a congenial gathering of similar people, in the communal style of assisted living. Staff are friendly, meals are provided, various types of group activities are usually available.

The difference is protection.

For starters, residents can't get out. If you've got a wanderer, this is huge. And if your loved one should later develop a wanderlust, it will be pleasantly but definitively stopped.

As with any facility, pay attention to the demeanor of the residents and staff. Does everybody seem to get along? Does staff pay attention to the residents throughout the day? What is the atmosphere at mealtime, and how are meals served? Are the communal areas pleasant and comfortable? How do they handle sundowning, the late afternoon state of confusion common to Alzheimer's patients?

Is there a carefully controlled, landscaped, outdoor space available to residents? Can the rooms be made to feel comfortable and homey with your loved one's own furniture?

You need to be extra vigilant on these subjects, because your loved one is no longer in a position to report any problems to you.

Memory care is expensive unless your loved one has significant resources or gold-encrusted insurance.

Finally, take really good care of yourself during this transition.

This is one of the hardest things anybody ever has to do for a loved one. Lean on your own support system. Pray. Seek comfort in your own private ways. Take a walk.

Remind yourself of the caregiving rewards you've used for yourself in the past. Dust them off and put them back into practice.

Permit yourself a period of denial and mourning, and don't feel guilty if that mourning carries a tinge of relief.

NINE
END OF LIFE ISSUES

T he end of life is steeped in euphemism, but the reality is that no matter what you call it, you are talking about death. Nobody likes to talk about death.

The impending death of a loved one is difficult under any circumstances. If you have been the primary caregiver, it is excruciating.

Everyone who is a part of this experience approaches it differently. Emotions run high. You are all facing the ultimate loss of control and nobody likes it one little bit.

Because this occurs on a continuum, even those who are most intimately involved may have very different ideas at any given moment. Your loved one is on the clearest path, slipping away from life. Beyond that, half a dozen dear ones will see it half a dozen ways.

Well-meaning friends will demonstrate the flaws in good intentions. People will absolutely say the wrong things, over and over again.

Your loved one's medical care team may never have been trained on how to speak about death. Until recently, the terminally ill were often not told that they were dying in order to "protect" them. Similarly uninformed family members didn't always have a chance to say goodbye.

Times have changed, but there still is no consistency from one doctor to another. The focus of most physicians is on *treatment*. Many believe their job is to continue suggesting treatments or clinical trials or other possibilities for prolonging life in anticipation of a miracle.

Miracles do happen, but they are rare.

Let's start by reviewing the Five Stages of Grief as first set forth by Elisabeth Kübler-Ross. We went through these earlier in the caregiving process (*see* CHAPTER SEVEN: CARING FOR THE CAREGIVER), because they apply to illness as well as to death.

- Denial
- Anger
- Bargaining
- Depression
- Acceptance

Keep in mind that while most people go through all these stages, they are not necessarily linear. Everyone involved may move back and forth from one to another, circle around to something they thought they were done with, or find themselves swamped simultaneously by several.

Please work extra hard to take care of yourself during the final stages of your loved one's life. You will sometimes feel that you need to be *doing* something, even when there is nothing to be done. You are also just as likely to find a dozen tasks and chores simultaneously drop on you.

Some caregivers take refuge in the mechanical aspects of management, while others find it impossible to concentrate on anything.

Know yourself. Accept that this will be hard, even if the anticipated passing is the sort sometimes referred to as "a blessing." If you need help, ask for it.

Understand that nobody will know what to say or do, so reach out specifically for whatever help you want or need. "Could you bring over a pizza?" is a perfect request. It's easy to make, easy to fulfill, and paves the way for the next request.

People do want to help. They just don't know how.

Make every effort to take your cues from the person at the center of this transition.

You may have always thought you knew exactly how your loved one would face death, and perhaps you were right. But it may also turn out differently.

Remember that while you confront a hole in your heart and an empty seat at the table, your loved one faces losing everything and everyone. People handle that awareness very differently.

ASPECTS OF CARE

The care of a dying patient is already moving along a treatment path, and initially this may remain unchanged.

At some point, however, you reach a fork in the treatment road. Will the patient continue to receive aggressive treatment aimed at thwarting the illness, cut back to less rigorous treatment, or decide to focus instead on quality of life, which may mean ending treatment altogether?

If the patient and caregiving team agree that the best approach is to fight the illness as hard as possible for as long as possible, very little change may occur at any point.

This approach is likely to eventually involve hospitalization and rehab in nursing homes, along with possible lengthy stays in intensive care. These settings relieve the caregiving team of much of the responsibility they have shouldered, placing it instead on medical personnel.

You also may see renewed efforts by family or friends to find clinical trials or unorthodox treatments, which the medical team won't necessarily support. The united family can shatter at this point unless everybody is on the same pathway.

With older patients, major surgery may be recommended simply because it is possible, despite the patient's age and condition. And also because Medicare will pay.

If the patient and caregiving team believe that the best approach is to ease back or end aggressive treatments, numerous practical matters will begin to change. If treatment has been exceptionally brutal or loaded with side effects, for example, just stopping it may represent definite improvement for the moment.

Palliative Care

Terminal patients may already be receiving forms of palliative care.

We spoke about palliative care earlier in SECTION FOUR: DI-
AGNOSIS, TREATMENT, AND MEDICATION, because it is often a part
of any patient's treatment. Palliative care is aimed at relieving
symptoms, discomfort, and stress. It is not part of the direct medical campaign against the underlying illness, and you can always
have one without the other.

Many people mistakenly think palliative care is synony-
mous with hospice. Not true. It is certainly *included* in hospice
care and sometimes added or enhanced.

Just as often, it precedes it.

Hospice

Hospice is a stage of treatment.

It's for people who are nearing the end of life. It offers a
compassionate and comfort-oriented course of care. Treatment
for the patient's illness stops, as do trips to the ER for matters
related to the illness. The focus changes to the patient and to
making the most of the time that remains.

The decision to enter hospice is made in consultation with
the medical team and requires medical authorization. The patient
or health care advocate must usually also agree.

Hospice has grown significantly in recent years. More than
half of all non-sudden deaths in the United States currently take
place in a hospice setting.

The customary criteria are scant possibility of recovery and
a likelihood that death will occur within six months. This does

not mean that the patient will be kicked out for exceeding the time limit, though a re-evaluation may occur.

Hospice does not represent giving up or failure—on the part of either patient or caregiving team. If that's how you have previously regarded hospice, please consider the many advantages before making any decisions.

Your loved one's care up to this point has been focused on medical needs. Hospice now adds the care of emotional and spiritual needs. Some of these may have been previously addressed, albeit as side elements of the illness.

A patient entering hospice is not just deciding how they wish to die. They are also deciding how they wish to *live* through their remaining days.

Very few people looking down the road at their own demise think that they'd really like to die in the hospital, hooked up to all kinds of equipment. But the wish for a miracle always lingers, and accepting hospice may seem to go against that.

In the past, dying patients were sometimes denied therapeutic levels of painkillers out of the misguided concern that they would become addicted to narcotics. These days, in situations where pain is a major issue, pain relief is often enhanced in hospice to keep the patient comfortable. The patient may even personally regulate the amount of medication to maintain an acceptable balance and level of pain relief.

It is important to understand that treatment for other, unrelated medical situations can continue. If somebody in hospice breaks a bone or develops an unrelated infection, these can and should be treated and may involve a trip to the ER.

Hospice may take place in a dedicated facility with a team that works exclusively with dying patients. In this case, you will be able to spend as much time as you want with your loved one, knowing that when you go home, someone will be available to provide needed assistance. A patient already in a nursing home can sometimes stay there through hospice.

Hospice may also occur at home, in familiar surroundings. This is closer to the scenario many people envision: loved ones gathered in a familiar bedroom, with music playing softly and a gentle breeze wafting through the open window.

Your hospice provider will bring in any necessary equipment—hospital beds, lifts, commodes, and so on. Home hospice does not, however, provide round-the-clock care. If your loved one requires that level of attention, you will need to recruit or hire caregiving help.

Wherever your loved one's hospice is based, you will be working with trained care providers who understand.

The hospice team may include different physicians and nurses than those you've been working with, as well as care managers, respite providers, counselors, and spiritual advisors. When the time comes, most hospice providers also offer grief counseling and grief support groups.

Any Medicare-certified hospice provider must offer both at-home and inpatient care, along with continuous care and respite care. Continuous care does not mean twenty-four-hour care but refers to periods of crisis when more than eight hours a day may be necessary.

Who pays?

Medicare and the VA both cover hospice—no surprise, since it is substantially less expensive than hospital care. Medicaid will cover the cost of room and board in a facility if the patient is already living in one. Most private insurance is also happy to go along because of both reduced expense and increased client satisfaction.

Get the particulars up front. And shop around if you can. Some hospice services may be better than others.

Find out if you have a choice in your area, or check with your insurance. If so, a little research will help enormously. This is something you probably don't want to farm out to secondary members of the caregiving team unless you know for sure they will have reactions you are likely to agree with.

Ask around. When you think about it, you probably know plenty of people with recent hospice experience. It doesn't need to be a close friend. Ask these people what they particularly liked—and particularly *didn't* like—about the service that they used. If there are complaints, see if they concern matters likely to bother you.

There is nothing wrong with doing some of this research secretly before you need it. Simply ask hypothetically. "We aren't there yet, but I'm wondering about hospice" is a perfect conversation starter, and you can follow the response in any way you choose.

Don't put it off too long, however. More than a third of hospice patients die within the first week.

How a family approaches hospice may depend more on personal attitudes than the specific realities of your loved one's situation. The decision to enter hospice can rip apart family unity. If one camp urges a continued fight and another embraces the concepts of care and comfort, you can find yourself in the midst of a major brouhaha.

Keep this in mind, however. People who have used hospice overwhelmingly come away with appreciation for the experience. Obituaries frequently request donations to hospice. And the single most commonly expressed regret is waiting too long.

DECISIONS

Handling practical matters may require a bit of detachment.

Variables may include: what kind of order the patient's affairs are in; who the family members are and where they live; the prognosis; religious beliefs; and the patient's attitude toward death.

Interspersed and tangled with these are the multiple other relationships among family and friends.

One thing you may notice right away is that people who were conspicuous by their absence during your loved one's illness will pop up with a lot of opinions on what *you* should be doing now. You are welcome to ignore them, particularly if you are the health care advocate.

Don't think you have to do everything all at the same time, but if you are having trouble concentrating, write things down.

What Does Your Loved One Want?

This is the question at the heart of everything you'll be doing. Maintain balance, of course. But always try to respect your loved one's wishes if you possibly can.

Is the Legal Paperwork in Order?

This is why we made such a big deal out of handling legal paperwork when everything was on a fairly even keel. If your loved one has signed paperwork for advance directives, durable power of attorney, and a will—you have one enormous burden lifted right away. If that's not the case, you need to deal with it *now*. Anything left until later has the potential to cause all kinds of problems down the road (*see* CHAPTER FIVE: THE PAPER JUNGLE). A will is particularly touchy in someone's final days, but you may be able to simplify this with online forms or Quicken WillMaker.

Nolo.com is loaded with proper, state-specific forms that you can download and work with immediately.

Who Decides What and When?

At every stage of illness, many decisions about medical care and treatment are made by the patient's physician. This involvement continues through decisions related to the impending loss of life.

If your loved one is in a position to make final decisions about their own care and treatment, respect those decisions.

But if the health care advocate is charged with this decision-making and the patient is unable to participate, everybody else needs to step out of the way. Make sure the patient's designated preferences are on file with doctors, hospitals, and any other care facility involved. Also carry hard copies with you and have them on your phone.

At some stage, the patient and physician may decide on a DNR (do not resuscitate, *see* CHAPTER FIVE: THE PAPER JUNGLE) order, which must be written by the doctor. This means exactly (and only) that if the patient stops breathing or their heart stops beating, health care personnel are not to perform CPR (cardio-pulmonary resuscitation).

A DNR does *not* mean that the patient won't be treated for other medical problems, such as a fall or an infection, or some entirely new medical issue.

In some states, a POLST (physicians order for life-sustaining treatment) can be created with even greater specificity.

If the patient can't participate in the creation and signing of either, it is part of the health care advocate's job.

DNRs should be posted on the refrigerator and bedside table where EMTs will automatically look for them. They are often hot pink to be obvious. Here's why that's important. Once the process of resuscitation is started, health professionals are trained to keep going. And if someone is inadvertently placed on life support, it can be very difficult to reverse that.

Yes, this does sometimes happen.

Life Support

Life support uses a combination of mechanisms and medications to supplement or replace a vital system that is not working well enough to sustain life. A patient on life support is likely to be in the ICU. This treatment is expensive.

Life support is intended to be a short-term substitution while affected organs heal and recover. It can also be used during such procedures as open-heart surgery. Usually, the patient is not conscious while on life support. It is not intended to continue indefinitely.

Life support can be discontinued when the physician and family agree to do so. This can get messy if family members disagree and the patient's wishes have not been clearly set out in advance.

Ending life support is not as simple as pulling a plug, though that is often how it's expressed, and you absolutely cannot pull that plug yourself. You may be certain that's what your loved one would want, but you could end up making your explanations from jail, facing homicide charges.

Physician-Assisted Suicide

This is an enormously complex and emotionally fraught topic. Under specific circumstances in a growing number of states, it may be possible for a doctor to prescribe medications that are likely to bring on death.

There is no longer a Hemlock Society, and Dr. Jack Kevorkian, imprisoned for assisting patients with suicide in the 1990s, is now dead himself. Further information is available at *compassionandchoices.org* and *finalexitnetwork.org*.

THE PERSONAL PART

Losing someone you love is really, really hard.

It becomes a part of your life in ways that you hadn't expected. It moves you in directions you may not want to go. It disrupts any parts of your life that might have remained comfortable. It does not adapt to your schedule or preferred timetable.

It creeps up on you and may remind you of its presence at awkward moments and in unanticipated places. You are never entirely removed from the process, even when you are technically away from it.

As you enter this stage, make sure that your own personal support system is firmly in place. If you've let it slide, get in touch with the people you lean on—family, personal friends, acquaintances who've experienced the same family illness, your faith community, support groups you've used while confronting the disease. (Use discretion here. Support groups where members are currently focused on fighting may not be helpful at this point.)

You don't need to ask for anything up front, but if people are forewarned that you are moving into new stages, they'll be ready when you look for support later. And you won't have to explain everything over and over again at that point.

Faith and Religion

The finality of death forces people to deal with their own attitudes and beliefs about death and afterlife. At some point in the process, everyone surrounding the patient will examine how death fits into their personal belief systems, even if they didn't want or intend to.

These thoughts can be confusing, confounding, and cathartic. Also exhausting.

You and your loved one may be a part of the same religion, perhaps even the same congregation within that faith. You might both reject organized religion or the role it has played in your lives and identify as agnostic or atheistic.

It's also entirely possible that you agree about nothing related to death and afterlife.

People change their minds on the subject as well. *There are no atheists in foxholes.* This isn't just a cliché in every war movie ever made. It's mostly true. When the subject is still abstract, it's easier to be cavalier.

But as the end approaches, so does a tendency to hedge one's bets. Just in case.

The person whose faith should be followed throughout this period is, of course, the patient. That doesn't mean that everybody else needs to convert or agree or abandon their own beliefs—just that the belief system of the dying person needs to be respected and prioritized.

Some people with intense religious beliefs may decide that your loved one must adopt those beliefs in order to do well in the afterlife. This situation becomes even rougher if *you* are the one whose beliefs are being challenged and your loved one does not appear interested in a deathbed conversion.

Two guidelines here: Nobody should pray directly over somebody who doesn't want to be prayed over. Nobody should quote scripture to somebody who doesn't want to hear it.

This doesn't mean that you can't be praying and quoting scripture to yourself, all the time if you feel the need. Just do it out of earshot of the patient.

You can and should follow your own faith during this impossible time. Seek personal guidance and counsel from the leaders of your own religion. If ever there were a time to immerse yourself in your beliefs, this is it.

Pray alone, with your spiritual leaders, with others in your faith community. Do what feels right for you, right now.

Beyond that, be gracious. Welcome any prayers, good thoughts, or spiritual offerings from anyone. In any way. In any religion.

Prayer offers solace and the possibility of feeling better, no matter what your beliefs.

Notifying People

This can be a tough one.

When do you tell somebody that the end is near for a relative or friend? If you wait until you yourself accept that awareness, it may be too late for others who wish to pay their respects to someone they are also losing.

So, try to step back a bit from this issue and consider it as a matter of logistics. Those who have been close throughout need to know, if they don't already. It's also useful to let people on the periphery know that the end may be approaching. This will simplify everyone's life and grief later.

Once again, the patient is at the heart of this process. Take your cues from your loved one.

On one end of this spectrum, some people who are dying and lucid feel a strong urge to reconnect one last time with folks who've meant a lot to them. They may also want to make things better with someone they've wronged, or to reconnect at least briefly with someone important to their past.

On the other end of the spectrum, somebody who feels and looks terrible may not want to see anybody at all. They may only be tolerating *you* because there's no choice. Some people who are dying don't want to talk to or deal with anybody, and even celebrities sometimes manage to keep it secret.

Do your best to honor those wishes. Explain later to anyone who feels slighted that it was not your decision and offer a slight shrug of your shoulders.

Meanwhile, get used to being on the tightrope in the middle. The patient comes first, but you can't automatically dismiss the needs and desires of others.

This is a good time to revisit the information you accumulated early on: lists of friends and associates, cards in the contacts box, folks who popped up in early stages of the health crisis. These are people you might want to get back in touch with, even if only by a gentle email that mentions declining health.

Distant relatives usually fit into this category. If you start with an email—individual to each person, even if it's the same text—you are also spared the need to repeatedly explain things, both now and later.

Estrangement

Has your loved one been estranged from someone who was once important? This can really matter at the end, and the other party might not even know that the clock is ticking. These situations are all different and personal, but keep in mind that if *you're* worried about death before resolution, it might also concern the aggrieved parties.

Bring up this person and situation as gently as possible, when the patient is at their best. Find out if they'd like to make peace or prefer to put everything behind them. It's their call, even if the other party has been in direct contact with you.

If you feel caught in the middle, however, don't squander time or energy on this battlefield. If the situation is becoming a problem, consult others who know your loved one well, or the patient's spiritual advisor. Then move cautiously away.

Be prepared to drop it, and perhaps to one day explain to the other party just what happened.

Feeling Guilty

Feeling guilty is such a standard feature of caregiving territory that you might not even notice how these feelings can change or intensify at the end of life.

This is no time for self-doubt. You have done the best you could with a horrible situation, and your best was good enough. Period. Repeat that to yourself as often as necessary until you believe it and use a mirror if necessary.

In any case, martyrdom is rarely an attractive quality.

Everybody makes mistakes. Everybody screws up now and then. Life is all about learning from what we may have done wrong and then moving on. Second-guessing *any* decisions at this point makes no sense and consumes energy you need for other things.

Sometimes it's the patient who feels guilty, for ignoring symptoms, or fighting treatment, or giving caregivers a hard time. Do your best to assure your loved one that none of that matters now and be equally forgiving to everyone else.

Falling Apart

At one point or another, most people facing the loss of a loved one will fall apart.

Crying, sobbing, screaming, pounding walls. Hating everything about what is happening. Yelling *WHY???* into the universe. This is a function of love, not of weakness. Roll with it.

Try to keep your own breakdowns away from the patient if you possibly can, but don't be afraid to let a tear slip or to show emotion. It's hard on them, too. You're all going through this loss together.

When the patient is the one who falls apart, don't pontificate. You just need to be there, holding your loved one if possible, mumbling assurances that it's all right. It's not all right, of course, but releasing pent-up emotions can be cathartic at a time when everyone really needs it.

After a while, you may find you've moved beyond the occasional breakdown, into a territory of constancy where you feel inconsolable and lost and furious all the time. If that's happening, consider talking things through with a grief counselor, or a therapist, or your spiritual advisor. These people deal with loss and grief repeatedly and may be able to help steady your feet on this rocky path.

Sometimes just being able to say the words out loud can help.

Saying Goodbye

People will want to say goodbye. There's no easy way around this.

You might even find your loved one surprising you with their own wishes here. Sometimes a shy wallflower and a social butterfly coexist—not just in the same garden, but also in the same person.

If your loved one is adamant about not seeing anybody, that's their call.

Just tell people that. Period.

Suggest cards or notes or emails that you can hand over or read to the patient. People might also provide something to share. At this juncture, the most useful gifts are those that you can eat up, drink up, or use up.

If the patient wants to have contact with others, find out who they want to see in person, who they'd like to call, and who they would definitely rather not see. Work from there. You may already be in contact with all of these people, or might have to do a little research to find somebody out of the past. If you hate this kind of contact work or tracking and somebody else in the caregiving circle is good with it—by all means delegate.

Schedule these meetings to conserve everybody's strength and keep them relatively brief. One-on-one is perfect. Small, obvious groups (Mahjong, church circle, fishing pals) work well. You set the agenda: time of day, length of visit, topics to discuss or avoid. If you find the process is wearing out the patient too much, reschedule or cut short without apology.

For relatives or friends who live afar and have limited means, paying for travel is a major consideration. Somebody who can only afford to come once might prefer to visit now rather than attend a later memorial service or funeral. Nobody needs to say this out loud.

Some people who are dying seem to wait until after a major family gathering: Thanksgiving, Christmas, Mother's Day. Others choose to throw their own "celebration of life" parties while they're able to attend.

There aren't any more rules at this point.

The End
You will be fine when the time comes. It's never been easy for anyone.

AFTERWARD
What happens after your loved one dies will depend a lot on your family and your religion.

Many faiths have strict and specific traditions related to death. If this applies to your family, your immediate steps are clear. Everybody knows what will happen and when and how. Choice is not an option and consistency is a relief and a comfort.

Where there is more flexibility, or no governing belief system, you have many possibilities. Perhaps too many. Take deep breaths and try to concentrate on what needs to be done *now.*

Arrangements
Unfortunately, you need to make a lot of decisions rather quickly, at a time when you are emotionally reeling. Perhaps the most wrenching are what we shall gently call the arrangements.

Some people make all their burial or cremation arrangements in advance, and in those cases you only need to follow their instructions. This is often prepaid, which is also good news.

You will usually need a funeral home and if there's a local choice and you're clueless, this is an awkward time for comparison shopping. Go with your instincts or recommendations from people you trust.

The services provided by a funeral home are not inexpensive, and they know you are vulnerable and not likely to quibble over much. If you or somebody close to your loved one is good at dealing with unctuous authoritarianism, that's who should be negotiating. And yes, negotiation is not inappropriate, particularly if expenses seem exorbitant. Ask questions. Get it in writing.

Cremation has moved into the mainstream in recent years, and more than half of all funeral arrangements in the United States are cremation rather than burial. This is an individual choice, and if your loved one didn't make it, the survivors can get into trouble over the issue. Clear this up and make a decision before you go any farther.

In some situations, families prefer to have a private burial or inurnment, with a celebration of life or other form of memorial sometime in the future. This can accommodate those who need to come from other places and also allows for a more celebratory feeling since time has passed.

Notifications

Notifications of the death of a loved one usually occur in a series of tiers, over a period of time. Speed is critical if a funeral or memorial service will occur quickly.

Begin with the nearest and dearest, those who were most likely aware that this was imminent. These close friends and family members should be told personally, and it's easiest to do this by phone. Exceptions are those who are elderly or frail or particularly sensitive. It's best to tell them in person.

You don't need to make these calls yourself, but somebody close to you and your loved one should. If there are branches of the family, call the obvious contact or the one you are closest to and ask them to spread the word among their own. The same is true for members of organizations, or work friends, or neighbors. Make it an information tree and let others worry about connecting the branches.

If there is going to be a service in the near future, you may want to wait until those details are clear and provide that information at the same time. That avoids a second round of calls. If you are requesting donations in lieu of flowers, it's useful to have the organization name and info.

Everyone will ask what they can do.

Before you get too deeply into this, figure out what things you *will* need and who's the best person for these jobs. Do you need somebody to go with you to the funeral home to make arrangements? Somebody for airport pickups? Somebody to design or write a memorial program? Set up a reception or meal after the services? Offer a spare bedroom to relatives from out of state?

Casseroles, flowers, and miscellaneous foodstuffs may begin to show up quickly. Some people keep funeral casseroles in the freezer, ready to go, and some fruit basket companies offer mourning assortments for overnight delivery.

It is not your responsibility to keep track of who brought what plate. If they want something back, people know to put on a sticker with their name and number.

Social Media

If you will be using social media to notify people of the passing or services, try to initially control the information. Who's putting up what, where, and when? You don't want people who should be personally notified to learn of this death because they had a couple of minutes to visit Facebook.

Recognize that once the information hits cyberspace, it is out there. You will quickly lose control.

If someone was active on social media, it's quite common for a relative to use their account to provide information. These accounts can usually be kept up or converted to memorial pages.

Obituaries

It is easiest to place formal newspaper obituaries through the funeral home. They know the appropriate contacts, protocols, deadlines, and fees. If you are notifying people so they can attend a service soon, you'll need to pull this information together in a hurry. That includes details like birthplaces and the correct spelling of relatives' names. You want to get this stuff right.

Obituaries used to run for free in newspapers as a public service, but they now mostly charge and are often quite pricey.

Photos cost extra. And speaking of photos, if you're going to use one, it doesn't have to be current. If there's a great picture from yesteryear that will make everyone smile in recognition, that's a good choice.

If your loved one was strongly connected to an organization, military group, or school, there is probably an easy online way to notify them for "In Memoriam" sections in newsletters or magazines.

Planning a Memorial

Some people who are dying take great pleasure in planning their own memorial services, down to hymn selections and who will or won't be asked to speak. If your loved one did this, then you only need to implement their wishes and peel yourself a grape from the fruit basket.

More likely, you may need to scramble a bit, because this is a skill set that you probably don't have.

If you are having the service at a funeral home, they will help manage most of the logistics.

If the service will be in a church or other religious institution, consult the appropriate personnel to secure times, officiants, soloists, organists, and ushers. Find out who gets paid what. If you have a choice in selecting music and the facility is willing, go with your loved one's favorites, including secular music.

Have somebody put together a brief biography for distribution and run it by the appropriate parties for accuracy. Print more than you think you'll need.

Arrange for any flowers you want to have at the service. Even when you specifically ask people not to send flowers, somebody usually will do so anyway. If you have a lot of flowers, perhaps the church will want to use some for upcoming services or can get them to residents of a nearby care facility.

If you wish memorial donations instead of flowers, you can designate an organization that was special to your loved one or simply ask for donations to the charity of the donor's choice. Put this request in the obituary and on social media.

If you intend to have some mourners attend a special reception or meal, try to delegate that entire process to somebody local and reliable. If that isn't possible, then keep it really simple.

The tone of a funeral, memorial service, or celebration of life can be whatever you choose (barring religious restrictions). A supplemental gathering where there aren't any rules might also occur sometime after more formal services.

People may go with a riverside picnic, a boat trip to sprinkle ashes, a weekend at the lake, a party at the local service or veterans lodge, or hanging out in somebody's backyard. Some of these celebrations feature a theme related to the loved one's personality or interests. Your options are wide open.

Death Certificates

The funeral home will usually arrange to get death certificates for you. These are official documents and you are likely to need more of them than you expect to. They are not cheap, but photocopies are not acceptable for many places that require them, starting with government agencies and financial institutions.

They can also take a while to arrive, another reason to order plenty up front. Later when you get down to business, you don't want to have to wait for a re-order from your state capital.

Legal Matters

You will need to take care of all kinds of technical and legal matters later, but for the most part nothing is likely to require your attention right away. This is particularly true if your loved one had their affairs in order. And if they didn't, now isn't the time to worry about it.

GRIEF

Grief is the price we pay for loving.

Everyone grieves differently, because every relationship is different. There is no right or wrong way to mourn, no matter what people may think or societal "norms" might suggest.

Someone you loved is gone. It's just that simple.

There's a hole in your heart, an empty seat at the table, a laugh unheard. You will find yourself healing over time, in different and unpredictable ways, but your relationship with the person who is gone now lives only in memory.

There is no timetable for grief. It changes over time, but it never entirely leaves you.

Your life will never be the same again. People talk about "getting over it" but you don't. The nature of your grief may change and mellow over time, but it doesn't go away.

Grief is lonely, even when there are many people grieving simultaneously.

If you are part of a culture with rigid ideas about grief, time-tables, and expected demonstrations of sorrow, your loss can be particularly intense because you are expected to keep it private and within acceptable guidelines.

Joseph R. Biden, a man who has known considerable personal loss, has often told groups of Gold Star family members and others in mourning: "One day, the thought of your loved one will bring a smile to your lips before it brings a tear to your eye."

He's right, though you may not believe it now.

Grief Support Groups

If your loved one was in hospice, you have probably already been dealing with grief counselors and clergy. Often these people also run grief support groups, and there may not be a charge, even if you were not involved with the sponsoring hospice organization.

Everybody is entitled to feel terrible, but if you're the sort of person who likes to talk things out, a structured setting can be an excellent idea. You may not need it for long, but it will probably help.

Compassionate Friends

Compassionate Friends (*compassionatefriends.org*) is the ultimate grief support group for parents who have lost their children. Volunteers know just what you are going through because they too have lost children, that most excruciating of all deaths. Many cities have groups that meet regularly, and these people really care.

Complicated Grief

Grief is normal and healthy and real, and people move through its stages at their own speed. However, some people are impacted far more severely than others, in a medically recognized condition called complicated grief.

Complicated grief can go on for years. The mourner remains intensely focused on the lost loved one, experiences boundless and continual sorrow, and is unable to function in ways that were previously not a problem.

This is for real. It is debilitating and can include physical symptoms. If you or someone in your family has gone for more than a year after a loved one's death and still seem to suffer deep and constant grief and pain, you should speak to your doctor or a mental health professional.

The Future

It might not feel like it right now, but there *is* a future. You will move into and through it the same way you went through your loved one's medical experiences and final days: putting one foot in front of the other, doing the best you can, and hoping for the best.

You are the caregiver for yourself now.

Give yourself time. Give yourself hope. Give yourself love.

RESOURCES

(Note: This list is designed to provide starting points for topics discussed and resources noted in Caregiving 101.*)*

Caregiving Information & Support

AARP – American Association of Retired Persons
aarp.org

CaringBridge – Private communication coordination
caringbridge.org

Family Caregiver Alliance
caregiver.org
800-445-8106

SibCare: The Trip You Never Planned to Take, by Taffy Cannon

Special Health Reports – Harvard Medical School
health.harvard.edu/special-health-reports

Diseases & Conditions

Alcoholics Anonymous
aa.org
800-839-1686

Alanon – For family members of alcoholics
al-anon.org
888-425-2666

Alzheimer's Association
alz.org
800-272-3900

American Cancer Society
cancer.org
800-227-2345

American Diabetes Association
diabetes.org
800-342-2383

American Heart Association
heart.org
800-242-8721

Circle of Care: A Guidebook for Mental Health Caregivers
National Alliance on Mental Illness
nami.org
800-950-6264

Dementia, Memory, and Brain Issues

American Brain Tumor Association
abta.org
800-886-2282

Caregiver's Guide to Understanding Dementia Behaviors
Family Caregiver Alliance
caregiver.org
800-445-8106

A Guide to Alzheimer's Disease
Harvard Medical School Special Reports
health.harvard.edu/special-health-reports

Improving Memory
Harvard Medical School Special Reports
health.harvard.edu/special-health-reports

My Stroke of Insight: A Brain Scientist's Personal Journey
Jill Bolte Taylor

The 36-Hour Day, by Nancy L. Mace and Peter V. Rabins

Practical Matters

DisposeMyMeds.org

HealthGrades: Find a doctor/doctor reviews/hospital ratings
healthgrades.com

Home Accessibility: 300 Tips for Making Life Easier, by Shelley Peterman Schwarz

Meals on Wheels
mealsonwheelsamerica.org
888-998-6325

National Prescription Drug Take-Back Days
takebackday.dea.gov

Nolo.com – State-specific legal paperwork
800-728-3555

Physicians' Desk Reference by Medical Economics – Drug information

ProPublica.org – Independent nonprofit newsroom

Quicken WillMaker – State-specific legal documents
nolo.com

Government Agencies

Healthcare.gov – Insurance through Affordable Care Act
800-318-2596

Medicaid.gov – Health coverage for low-income people
800-633-4227

Medicare.gov – Health coverage for older people
800-633-4227

VA.gov – Health coverage for military veterans
800-698-2411

End of Life
Compassionate Friends – Support for parents who have lost children
compassionatefriends.org

Hospice Foundation of America
hospicefoundation.org
800-854-3402

National Hospice and Palliative Care Organization
caringinfo.org
800-658-8898

On Death and Dying, by Elizabeth Kübler-Ross

POLST: Physician Orders for Life Sustaining Treatment
polst.org
202-780-8352

ALSO BY THE AUTHOR

SibCare: The Trip You Never Planned to Take

*****

Convictions: A Novel of the Sixties

A Pocketful of Karma

Tangled Roots

Class Reunions are Murder

Mississippi Treasure Hunt (young adult)

Guns and Roses: A Modern Mystery Set in Colonial Williamsburg

The Tumbleweed Murders (completed for the late Rebecca Rothenberg)

Open Season on Lawyers

Paradise Lost

Blood Matters

Beat Slay Love (with Kate Flora, Lise McClendon, Katy Munger, and Gary Phillips)

*****

Written as Emily Toll:

Murder Will Travel

Murder Pans Out

Fall into Death

Keys to Death

ABOUT THE AUTHOR

Taffy Cannon is the author of *SibCare: The Trip You Never Planned to Take*. She has also written fourteen mysteries, an Academy-Award-nominated short film, and *Convictions: A Novel of the Sixties*. As a *Jeopardy!* contestant, she once correctly wagered everything on a Women Writers Daily Double. She lives with her husband in Southern California, where she gardens year-round and was named Citizen of the Year for service to her local library.

www.TaffyCannon.com and *www.SibCare.org.*